P9-BBP-510

How To Control Your Allergies

by Robert Forman, Ph.D.

Larchmont Books
Atlanta, Georgia

Eighth Printing:	*January, 1984*
Seventh Printing:	*August, 1983*
Sixth Printing:	*May, 1983*
Fifth Printing:	*October, 1982*
Fourth Printing:	*February, 1982*
Third Printing:	*March, 1981*
Second Printing:	*May, 1980*
First Printing:	*June, 1979*

HOW TO CONTROL YOUR ALLERGIES

Copyright © Larchmont Books, 1979

ISBN 0-915962-29-2

Printed in the United States of America

LARCHMONT BOOKS
*6255 Barfield Rd.
Atlanta, Ga. 30328*

Contents

A DUAL DEDICATION

I. Dedicated to the various general practitioners and internists, the three eye, ear, nose and throat specialists, and the allergist whom I consulted over the years. If any one of them had known of and employed the information contained in this book, it would never have been written.

II. Dedicated to all the doctors mentioned herein, whose lonely pioneering has contributed so much to the welfare of their patients and the establishment of the exciting field of Clinical Ecology.

Foreword

PROFESSOR FORMAN's extensive background in the field of sociology and his personal experience with severe forms of internal allergy make him highly qualified to write this book. He is in the unique position of being able to present intricate problems of bio-ecologic medicine from the viewpoint of both the patient and academician.

As a patient, Dr. Forman has experienced many of the discomforts and frustrations that his readers or their loved ones have had. In this well written book, he shares with others the medical enlightenment that led to his recovery and the happiness that others may also achieve. He has augmented his knowledge by studying the important medical literature on this subject, and he has spent many hours with me and my staff as a visiting professional colleague at The Alan Mandell Center for Bio-Ecologic Diseases.

With the kind permission of a number of my patients, who want to help others by sharing their experiences with them, Dr. Forman had a number of excellent opportunities to observe how I diagnose patients suffering from many forms of complex bio-ecologic disorders. He was present in my consultation room as I reviewed many facets of their past medical histories in great detail, and he knows how I selected a series of symptom-duplicating provocative sublingual tests to identify environmental offenders that affected each patient. He understands how a comprehensive individualized program of physiologically sound nondrug management is formulated to treat every aspect of each susceptible patient's physical or mental disorder resulting from the combined effects of environmental factors and the patient's overall nutritional state.

I am very pleased to write the Foreword to *How to Control Your Allergies* because this is a positive, helpful—and hopeful—book. I am certain that some of Dr. Forman's readers may, for the first time, begin to realize the importance of allergy, proper nutrition and a clean health-sustaining indoor and outdoor environment. It will be possible for many readers to experience a new outlook on life by changing their eating and working habits and life style. They will learn more about their environment, about sociology and how they themselves can exert considerable influence on their own destiny with respect to good mental health and physical well being.

This book is an excellent introduction to the environmentally and biologically oriented holistic approach to many chronic and recurrent forms of physical and mental illness caused by previously unrecognized allergies and allergy-like disorders. Dr. Forman presents a common sense and physiologically sound way to better health to many of the "forgotten people" whose illness is not understood or being properly treated by the currently employed methods of modern medicine and psychiatry. My colleague, Dr. Harris Hosen, coined this term to describe the millions of patients who believe that they have been forgotten and have given up hope that the nature of their illness would ever be understood well enough so that they could recover.

To better appreciate the fundamental importance of bio-ecologic influences that profoundly affect the quality and length of human life, the reader should see himself in relation to the natural scheme of things. First, the reader should be aware of the importance of the physical and mental health of one's parents during the biologically significant period of time prior to his or her conception. Environmental substances that are ingested and inhaled by the parents of each human being have a direct effect on the composition, development and quality of the sperm and the fertilized egg from which that individual subsequently arises. The egg and sperm are influenced by the biochemical reactions associated with normal body functions, daily activities and the various mental and physical stresses that parents experience.

Throughout pregnancy there is an uninterrupted sequence of exposures to a complex group of essential nutrients and numerous biologically active environmental agents—ecologic factors—which have far reaching consequences on the developing fetus. Prenatal (intrauterine) exposures have permanent effects that are reflected in that individual's postnatal health for his entire life.

The moment our postnatal lives begin, we start an unending series of interaction with many types of environmental substances. We come into contact with them continuously during a life time of eating, drinking, breathing and participating in various daily activities. Numerous kinds of biologically active materials from our surroundings enter the body through our lungs and gastrointestinal tracts. They are transported throughout our bodies by means of the circulatory system. Every cell, tissue, organ and system—including the brain and the nervous system—is repeatedly exposed to this highly diverse group of reactive natural and synthetic factors from the world around us.

Some of the substances that we interact with cause cellular injury that may result in forms of physical or mental illness. We become sick because we ingest and inhale natural and man-made substances that are not compatible with our biologically and biochemically unique

7

makeup which is genetically determined and modified by our nutritional state and a life time of exposure to various toxic substances.

In their early stages, an overwhelming majority of these environmentally induced disorders of body and mind are completely reversible biologic disturbances. In many instances they can be controlled (prevented or cured) by eliminating or reducing exposure to the illness-causing factor(s). Physiologic and nutritional treatments will increase the affected individual's resistance by decreasing his internal state of susceptibility that predisposes him to become sick from contact with offending environmental substances.

A large proportion of our normal intake of 1,000 nutritionally inadequate, vitamin and mineral deficient meals a year consists of modified, processed, packaged, flavored, colored, polished, refined, preserved, waxed, bleached, de-germed, de-braned, extended, contaminated and agro-chemically poisoned foods. Our fruit, vegetables and grains are grown in soil of poor quality and the health and quality of our poultry and livestock leaves much to be desired.

In addition to the ingestion of these 1,000 unnatural, damaged and dangerous meals annually, many individuals are also exposed to those often irresistible between-meal snacks or the large quantity of tidbits that are consumed during years of midnight raids on the pantry or the refrigerator. These temporarily satisfying and seminutritious dietary excursions may include sugar-loaded junk foods and in many instances this pattern of compulsive eating is a manifestation of a completely unrecognized state of addictive food allergy that Dr. Forman will unmask for you in this book.

Before a susceptible individual reaches the chronic and addictive stage of a bio-ecologic illness of body or mind, there may be a series of acute episodes of his or her patient-specific allergic disorder(s) that usually are of relatively brief duration. Many people who have been indisposed by such masquerading ailments are frequently misdiagnosed by themselves or their physicians as being victims of a "24-hour virus" or psychologic and social stresses. Millions of patients are consulting with their physicians to find the cause of virus-like illnesses, mild to moderate "emotional upsets" or psychosomatic disorders that are, in fact, unsuspected and unrecognized allergic and allergy-like reactions to certain foods, beverages, airborne allergens and environmental chemical substances. Unfortunately, the majority of these patients and their doctors do not yet understand the essential nature of these physical and mental problems and how to treat them and that is Dr. Forman's reason for writing this book.

With every breath we take we may inhale one or several of the countless and possibly dangerous airborne chemicals that many of us appear to be able to cope with at present. But we are becoming more and more intimidated by this endless stream of potential offenders that are produced by our modern chemical technology. Writing in the July 13, 1978 issue of *New Scientist,* Dr. Robert Lewin reports that there are an estimated 100,000 chemicals in more or less common usage in the Western industrialized world. And each year several thousand more are added to the list. Such a profusion of man-made substances is a matter of great concern to every citizen as well as to the ecologist and carcinogenist (cancer specialist). Neither man nor his planet has had any previous experience in dealing with this abundance of new and potentially dangerous chemical agents.

What is especially alarming to environmentalists is that many of these chemicals contaminate our daily food, air and water supply and they have not been sufficiently tested for long-term effects to insure that they are unquestionably safe for all of us. And this danger is augmented by the fact that two or more of these chemicals may combine to create newer and even more harmful substances. The possible combinations of the current arsenal of inadequately tested chemicals is mind-boggling and runs into the millions.

To this ever-growing list of man-made chemicals, we must add the countless natural allergens that have plagued human beings for hundreds of thousands of years: foods, pollens, molds, bacteria, dusts, feathers, animal danders and insects.

With so many actual and potential offending agents present in the environment, is it any wonder that more and more professionals and laymen alike have become deeply concerned about these threats to human health? Some presently encountered chemical agents are regarded as being serious threats to the continued existence of our species. People are becoming involved with their environment, with better nutrition, with human ecology and with how these intertwining influences affect our physical, mental and emotional health. As the clinical ecologists and their followers became more enmeshed in this complex subject, they soon began to realize the great extent to which allergy, addiction and allergy-like sensitivity to natural and man-made substances are responsible for widespread physical and mental illness and, in fact, may undermine the health and activity of whole societies.

As a sociologist, Dr. Forman is in the enviable position of being qualified to assess certain aspects of the impact of widespread allergy-based medical, surgical and psychiatric problems that occur in people who become reactive to foods, beverages, inhalants and environmental chemical agents that enervate millions of people each year. I believe that his profound statement will stimulate the interest of many colleagues who are not acquainted with the potentials of bio-ecologically oriented medicine and psychiatry.

The book is a welcomed addition to the literature on bio-ecologic disorders. It carefully shows the reader how to begin to control and perhaps eliminate the reversible disorders of body and mind that are due to allergy, addiction and susceptibility to the modern chemical environment.

MARSHALL MANDELL, M.D., D.A.B.A.I., F.A.C.A.
New Canaan, Conn.
January, 1979

Dr. Mandell is a former assistant professor of pediatric allergy of the New York Medical College; Medical Director for the New England Foundation for Allergic and Environmental Diseases, Norwalk, Conn.; author of "Dr. Mandell's 5-Day Allergy Relief System; Allergy, The Unrecognized Cause of Physical, Mental and Psychosomatic Illness," Thomas Y. Crowell Division, Harper & Row, 1979.

CHAPTER 1

Food Allergy: Medicine's Stepchild

THE FACT YOU are reading this book probably means that you suspect that you or someone close to you may be affected by allergies. Everyone has heard of them and most likely knows someone who suffers from allergy. To the outsider the allergy victim is a comic character whose troubles can draw laughs in movies or on television. The entertainment media also usually show allergy sufferers as being odd people, their lives and personalities warped by their need to protect themselves from the cause of their troubles. While allergy may very well affect its victims in this way, there certainly is nothing funny about it to the person so afflicted.

Allergy is probably the most frequently unrecognized physical condition in America, with the majority of those affected by it not even realizing that their troubles are due to it. In earlier years a number of studies were made in order to estimate just how prevalent allergy was. Groups or whole communities numbering in the hundreds or thousands were screened for allergy symptoms. The studies showed a considerable amount of agreement in finding that about 50% of the people had recognizable allergy symptoms.[1] Considering that investigators inquired about only the more obvious symptoms and that not all indications of allergy were recognized at the time the true figure must be somewhat above half of the population. For the United States this amounts to more than 100 million people!

Fortunately, the majority of those affected by allergy do not suffer seriously from the condition. But even a minority out of a total of 100 million can be a large number of people! Two allergists writing in the 1970's also put the figure at over 100 million, believing that some "20 million suffer with allergies severe enough to require serious attention."[2] This minority is thus about equal to the whole population of California and is almost three times the number of residents of New York City. This certainly is a large quantity of allergy sufferers!

Conventional Allergists vs. Clinical Ecologists

If allergy is so common why is not more attention paid to it? One reason has already been mentioned, that the majority of cases are relatively mild or periodic so that they do not involve great or prolonged discomfort. Another is that, in many instances, even serious ones, the trouble is not recognized as being due to allergy but may be attributed by doctor and layman alike to other causes. This can lead to extensive surgery, prolonged psychiatric therapy, elaborate medication or expensive diagnostic procedures.

One allergist described the situation this way: "Often the tragic result is that allergic patients undergo operations for appendicitis, gallbladder trouble or other intestinal ailments when the trouble really is allergy. These unfortunate people are the victims of a mistaken diagnosis. A doctor properly trained to recognize the symptoms of allergy might easily have saved them from pain, great cost, and waste of time."[3]

A colleague of mine recently underwent about $700 of diagnostic tests as medical school doctors tried to locate the cause of a variety of symptoms, including muscle pains, digestive upsets so severe they woke him up in the middle of the night, and a feeling of weakness and lack of energy. They mentioned the possibility of various uncommon scary diseases but could find nothing conclusive. When, at my suggestion, he tried experimenting with his diet to see if foods played a part, he quickly found that all his troubles came from a sensitivity to milk, which he of course then stopped drinking. One day shortly after this he popped his head in my office to tell me, "I was able to ride my bicycle today for the first time in more than a year." And another time he stopped by gleefully reporting, "I painted my garage over the weekend. A few weeks ago I could hardly hold a brush."

This failure of many doctors to recognize the importance of allergy and to consider it a serious possibility in making diagnoses comes, strangely enough, from a problem within the field of allergy itself. The majority of allergists, particularly those who are teaching in university medical schools, tend not to be interested in allergy to foods, not to look for it as often, to use only a limited number of methods in trying to detect it, and to downplay the importance of food allergy generally. I shall call these the conventional allergists.

A small minority of allergists, though, over the past several decades has become interested in food allergy, has investigated it extensively and has developed and used a wider variety of methods for detecting food allergy in their patients. We can call them the food allergists. Many of these same doctors, however, have also gone further than the conventional allergists in identifying and developing means for testing allergic susceptibility to chemical substances in food and in the air. Their work in the area of both foods and chemicals has attracted the attention of medical specialists in other areas, who have found it helpful and relevant for the problems they have been encountering. Together, they have been developing a new field of medicine which is coming to be called *clinical ecology*.

This specialty concerns itself with an individual's environment—the food in it that one eats, the home, the place of work, the neighborhood—any of which might contain substances the person is sensitive to and thereby cause trouble for him or her. Clinical ecology emphasizes identifying and minimizing the effect of environmental exposures that can be harmful to a person rather than just using drugs to alter the body processes or to cover up symptoms.[4] As one clinical ecologist points out, there are many effective headache remedies available today, and a person who takes such a remedy may have the headache go away quickly but will not learn what caused the headache.[5] Similarly, an anti-histamine may stop a runny nose.

So the ability to get relief in five minutes discourages both doctor and patient from really digging out the cause of the trouble. But if the problem can be solved in this way, then why not do so? Because, the clinical ecologists emphasize, using drugs to trick the body into an absence of symptoms creates more serious problems in the long run. The allergic condition which caused the symptoms does not go away with cover-up treatment. As we will see in a later chapter, continued exposure to a substance to which a person is allergic creates stress within the body and eventually leads to serious illness when the body's adaptive mechanism becomes exhausted.

Clinical ecologists have found that allergy to foods is much more prevalent than has been believed and that it is the cause of many more illnesses than has been recognized by conventional medicine. Table I lists some of the illnesses or symptom syndromes which have been found to be caused in at least some cases by allergy, as indicated by the fact that they have been successfully treated through

15

Table 1. Some Symptoms or Conditions That Have Been Found to be Caused by Allergy

I. Appearance and skin
    1. acne
    2. canker sores
    3. dark circles under eyes
    4. dermatitis
    5. eczema
    6. hives
    7. itching
    8. pale color not due to anemia
    9. psoriasis
    10. skin reddening
II. Headache
    11. various kinds including migraine
III. Eye Conditions
    12. conjunctivitis
    13. eye pain
    14. periods of blurred vision
    15. sensitivity to light
    16. tearing
    17. temporary refractive changes
IV. Ear Conditions
    18. hearing loss
    19. infections
    20. inflammations
    21. Menière's syndrome
    22. noises in the ear
    23. repeated ear trouble
V. Cardiovascular
    24. angina
    25. high blood pressure
    26. irregular heartbeat
    27. low blood pressure
    28. rapid pulse
VI. Gastrointestinal

29. constipation
30. diarrhea
31. gall bladder pains
32. gas
33. gastric ulcer
34. gastro-intestinal bleeding
35. heartburn
36. hemorrhoids
37. indigestion
38. mucous colitis
39. nausea
40. nervous stomach
41. pains or cramps
42. spastic colon
43. vomiting

VII. Respiratory
44. asthma
45. chronic rhinitis
46. coughing
47. frequent "colds"
48. hay fever
49. mouth breathing
50. nosebleeds
51. postnasal discharge
52. sinusitis
53. stuffy nose
54. wheezing

VIII. Urological
55. bedwetting
56. frequent night urination
57. frequent urination
58. painful or difficult urination

IX. Muscular-skeletal
59. arthritis
60. joint pains
61. muscle cramps
62. muscle pains and aches
63. muscle spasms

64. muscle weakness

X. Mental-behavioral

65. anxiety
66. delusions
67. depression (including psychotic)
68. dizzy spells
69. drowsiness
70. epilepsy
71. floating sensations
72. general fatigue
73. hallucinations
74. hyperactivity
75. insomnia
76. irritability
77. learning disorders
78. minimal brain dysfunction
79. nervousness
80. periods of confusion
81. phobias
82. poor concentration
83. poor memory
84. poor muscle coordination
85. restlessness
86. schizophrenia
87. sleeps at inappropriate times

Sources: Arthur F. Coca, M.D., *The Pulse Test,* ARC Books, New York, 1959, p. 17; William G. Crook, M.D., *Your Child and Allergy,* Professional Books, Jackson, Tenn., 1973, p. 20; Marshall Mandell, M.D., Abstract of presentation to convention of the International Academy of Metabology, March 23, 1973, Table II; William H. Philpott, M.D., *Ecological Medicine Manual,* Oklahoma City, Okla., 1975 (mimeographed) pp. 2–3; Herbert J. Rinkel, M.D., Theron G. Randolph, M.D., and Michael Zeller, M.D., *Food Allergy,* Charles C. Thomas, Springfield, Ill., 1951, passim.

88. sleeps too little
89. sleeps too much
90. tension-fatigue syndrome
91. unsteadiness
XI. Other
92. abnormal body odor
93. diabetes
94. excessive sweating
95. general weakness
96. hypoglycemia
87. night-sweating
98. overweight
99. underweight
100. virus infections

detecting and managing patients' allergies. The ultimate statement about possible effects of allergy comes from two specialists in the field who wrote: "It has now been accepted as factual that allergy may be a potential cause of any medical condition."[6] An English doctor refers to food and chemical allergy as ecological illness and estimates that, of all illness, 30% is due completely to allergy, 30% is partly attributable to allergy, and only the remaining 40% is unrelated to allergy.[7]

It is not uncommon for an allergic person to have several symptoms or conditions all due to allergy. One woman, for example, had migraine, colitis, attacks of dizziness and fainting, abnormal tiredness, and indigestion.[8] Another patient had colitis, gall bladder pains, chronic rhinitis, headache, joint and muscle pains, irregular heartbeat, and painful urination as well as such "psychological" conditions as dizzy spells and mental confusion.[9] One proof that these symptoms were all caused by allergy is that when the guilty foods were detected and avoided in the diet all the symptoms cleared up at about the same time.

But, you may be wondering, doesn't this ignore all that is known about the importance of viruses and bacteria as causes of illness? Clinical ecologists do not deny that these agents can cause disease, but they point out that the health of the body tissues and consequent ability to fight off germs will be poorer for the person suffering from allergic reactions. Dr. Lendon Smith has found that patients who had frequent ear and kidney infections no longer got them after their allergies were treated.[10] In other words, the viruses and bacteria will be around, but whether the person succumbs to them will depend upon his overall health and resistance. As Dr. Arthur F. Coca said, "You don't catch colds—you eat them."[11]

This food allergy pioneer, whose work supplied many of the items listed in Table 1 wrote that the proof for his claims was that the symptoms disappeared after the allergies were detected and treated by eliminating the guilty foods from the diet and they reappeared if the foods were again eaten.[12] Other food allergists have used the same standards. No one claims that allergy is the only cause of these conditions. Indeed, that is why allergy is so mystifying and elusive. It can be responsible for symptoms which can also be produced by other causes. Fortunately, at least with food allergy, once one knows some of the basic principles of how it works, it can be relatively easy to see if it is the culprit in a particular case. There will be more on this later.

Yet, conventional allergists are reluctant to grant that food allergy can cause so many difficulties. The authors of one medical textbook, for example, while conceding that food allergy "appears to be relatively common in the community at large," go on to warn that "the allergist should avoid the pitfalls of overdiagnosing food allergy."[13] They believe that: "Many people would rather attribute their complaints to food allergy than to a less acceptable but correct diagnosis of psychoneurosis. . . . Ultimately, the allergy program fails to give relief, and such a fixation to being sensitive to foods is developed that subsequent psychotherapy is most difficult."[14]

While such a caveat might be expected to come from psychiatrists or internists, it is surprising to find allergists downplaying their own field. Minimizing the importance of one's specialty is certainly rare not only in medicine but also in the world at large. One wonders if the allergists who made the above statement had really used all possible methods to detect the guilty foods; if we may judge from the evidence in their book, they did not. We shall see later that there are a number of effective methods for detecting food allergies that are not commonly used and why they have not been.

Hirschfeld describes the 19th century physicians who "cloaked their ignorance of what we call allergic reactions and their causes by diagnosing them as hysteria or neuroses."[15] Indeed, modern clinial ecologists are reversing the order of the sequence. Instead of saying that complaints believed by the patient to be due to allergy are really psychiatric, they are showing that a number of psychiatric conditions are caused by allergy. Following the traditional views described above, the allergy patient would be referred to a psychiatrist only to find in many cases that the psychotherapy was not helpful. The psychiatrist could maintain that he really was right but that the patient was exhibiting resistance, had a fixation, was repressing, etc. and the patient had no recourse. Unless allergy is definitely ruled out, I will side with the patient.

Dr. William B. Sherman, the author of a medical text which listed more than 50 conditions that had been ascribed to allergy by food allergists, gave as one reason for not accepting most of these as allergy-caused: "Most of the symptoms attributed to allergy have been purely subjective and of a neurasthenic type."[16] Certainly a "tired draggy feeling" would be a classic example of a type of neurasthenic complaint, yet this is exactly what a major textbook on food allergy reported as one of the most common of allergy symptoms.[17] Most doctors would probably view such a complaint as a psychiatric one, particularly after giving a battery of lab tests and getting no indication of physical malfunctioning. The authors of the latter text also take issue with a psychosomatic explanation for "allergy as well as in other chronic unexplained illnesses," maintaining that it "is all too frequently a matter of expediency on the part of the physician."[18]

Clinical ecologist Marshall Mandell has described a number of cases of patients who had undergone psychotherapy without success, sometimes for years, whose difficulties were due to allergy.[19] One man, for example, suffered from mental confusion, severe fatigue, nervous tension, and frequent "virus infections." "A psychiatric consultant had concluded that emotional stress was the underlying cause of the recurrent and disabling illness; he informed the patient that his poor health was due to lowered resistance which in turn, was the consequence of unresolved mental problems that required a psychotherapeutic approach." He turned out to be allergic to a number of foods in his diet. By avoiding these he remained well without need for medication or further treatment, a result which could not have been brought about by a lifetime on the psychiatric couch.

Conventional allergists have also been skeptical of allergy as a cause of gastrointestinal complaints[20] yet these are frequently cleared up by the avoidance of the foods to which a patient is allergic. One clinical ecologist, Dr. Richard Mackarness, discusses ulcerative colitis as an example of a serious and sometimes even fatal disease which frequently is due to food allergy, the prime offender being milk. Treatment may involve surgical removal of all or part of the colon with a new opening being made in the abdomen for the release of food wastes, which, in the words of Mackarness are "mutilating operations that can be psychologically devastating to the victim."[21]

While the food most commonly found to cause ulcerative colitis is milk, other foods sometimes are responsible also. Mackarness cites studies showing that when milk and milk products were removed from patients' diets their condition improved and when milk was introduced again another attack of the disease resulted. Despite the fact that the evidence for this goes back at least to 1942, it is not uncommon to hear of colitis patients who have been told by their doctors to follow a milk diet. Mackarness considers ulcerative colitis a good example of an illness which is viewed by most doctors as "psychosomatic (caused by the mind influencing the body)," but is "really somatopsychic (caused by the body influencing the mind and behavior)."[22]

Arthritis is one disease that has not generally been considered as psychosomatic; neither has it been one which doctors have viewed as caused by allergy in even some cases. The Arthritis Foundation has been reluctant to accept the view that one's diet may influence the course of arthritis. Yet, food allergists early found cases of arthritis that appeared to be caused by allergy. One group of food allergists reported that they found that arthritis symptoms were relieved through control of allergy and added: "Many cases of this type are seen in the practice of allergy." The doctors reported that "we have been able to produce arthritis attacks at will by feeding specific foods."[23] When their patients avoided the foods to which they were allergic, they did not have arthritis attacks when there were changes in the weather.[24]

Thus, food allergists point to medical conditions ranging all the way from behavior through alterations in or malfunctioning of the body organs to structural changes in the bones themselves as being caused at least part of the time by allergy. But most conventional allergists, which means the great bulk of all allergists, refuse to accept this, preferring to limit their scope to the few diseases classically associated with allergy.

Allergy and Immunology

How this whole situation came about is not too hard to see in terms of the development of the field of allergy, which took place almost all in the present century. Even the word allergy was not coined until 1906. Earliest observations and research in the field were concerned mainly either with human diseases like hay fever, caused by airborne proteins such as pollen, or with the reactions of laboratory animals to injections of such apparently innocent substances as serums and egg white. While the first injection of a particular substance into an animal would produce no observable response, the same material injected a few days later would result in a reaction. In some cases, particularly with guinea pigs, it could be strong enough to be fatal.

Both hay fever and the reaction of the animals to the second injection (the reaction is called anaphylactic shock) of a substance were traced to the same physiological mechanism, the operation of the immune system. This is the system that enables us to fight off bacteria and causes the body to reject, say, a skin graft supplied by another person. As described by Dr. Ben Feingold: "Allergy cannot be defined without a consideration of the nature of immunity. Immunity involves all the mechanisms concerned with the protection of the individual against the assult of foreign substances. A foreign substance is any material which the body does not recognize as *self,* i.e., a part of itself.... Since allergy is a variation of the basic immune mechanism, a discussion of allergy is actually a

24

consideration of the mechanism of immunity."[25]

This means that the same mechanism which protects you from germs may also give you your hay fever. It also explains why the laboratory animals had no reaction to their first exposure to an injected foreign substance. It fell on unfertile soil. However, the injection was quickly recognized by the body as being foreign—not part of itself—and the immune mechanism went to work making antibodies and preparing itself to fight off the invader if it should come again. This is the same process that makes vaccination both possible and necessary.

On our first exposure to a certain type of bacteria, we are not prepared to resist it and so we get sick. A vaccination, on the other hand, exposes us to a very weak or dead strain of the bacteria so that it is not strong enough to make us sick but does prepare us to resist the regular bacteria if we are later exposed to them. Our first contact gets our immune system to produce antibodies to the bacteria so that it can respond quickly enough to keep us from getting sick upon the second exposure. But under some circumstances the immune systems of both man and animal can over-respond, which is what happens in the cases of both hay fever and anaphylactic shock. Hay fever is an over-reaction of the immune system to a substance (pollen) to which it was exposed before and which it recognizes as foreign.

It was early observed that injection of a small amount of a substance to which a person was allergic would produce a reaction on the skin at the site of the injection, which led to skin tests as a means of allergy detection. Treatment of allergy then became a matter of a series of injections of minute amounts of the offending material so that the patient would gradually lose his oversensitivity to it, a process called desensitization. The body learned to tolerate it and the patient's symptoms were relieved.

25

By 1926 the "descriptive term *allergy* was redefined immunologically."[26] In other words, allergy came to be defined only in terms of conditions related to the body's immune system. Immunity and allergy both stem from the same mechanism. "Those reactions which appear to benefit the individual are considered manifestations of immunity, those that are harmful, manifestations of allergy."[27] But most food allergies, while sometimes producing classic allergy symptoms, involve other body mechanisms which are not as well understood. Skin tests for it do not work well and desensitization shots are ineffective.

What knowledge there is of food allergy indicates that it is a matter of a lack of or malfunctioning of enzymes in the digestive process. However, to the conventional allergist this is all the more reason for excluding food sensitivity reactions from even the definition of allergy. One modern conventional textbook stated: "The recent discovery of enzyme mechanism in many such cases [of food allergy] make it increasingly important to reserve the term 'allergy' for cases of definitely proved or reasonably positive immunologic mechanisms. Use of the term in a broader sense destroys its scientific value."[28]

Thus from this standpoint it is incorrect to even speak of food allergy and some other term should be employed to refer to sensitivities and conditions relating to food. According to this view, allergy equals immunology. One recent allergy textbook is titled *Clinical Aspects of Immunology* and does not concern itself with food allergy in its more than 1,700 pages.

Although Dr. Ben Feingold, as we shall see later, recognizes the importance of food in producing both behavioral and physical symptoms, he nevertheless reserves the concept of allergy just for conditions relating to the immune system, and writes not of food allergy, but of "adverse reactions" to food, believing that these may be either immunologic or nonimmunologic in nature.[29] As both popular usage and that of many doctors includes food sensitivity as part of allergy, whether a function of the immune system or not, I will use the term food allergy in the broad sense, recognizing that the majority of cases of food allergy are probably not involved with the immune system.

Whereas conventional allergy practice concerned with inhaled pollens, etc. rests, as one textbook put it, on "immunologic principles soundly based on proved facts...much of the study of food allergy is empirical practice with no relation to basic science and no knowledge of the pathogenic mechanisms involved."[30] This means that conventional allergists reject food allergy because they don't know how it works.

The fact that the ecological allergists can point to patients whose symptoms were alleviated cuts no mustard with the conventionals. When the latter ask what caused the symptoms, the ecologists have to answer that they really don't know, but that they found through experimenting with the patient's diet that his symptoms went away when they had him stop eating rutabagas or whatever. Furthermore, they say that using this approach enables them to correct not just a runny nose or hives but any of the scores of conditions mentioned earlier.

This is all too much for the conventional allergists. The author of the textbook quoted above also wrote: "It was the later expansion of the concept that made many conservative internists and pediatricians skeptical of the words 'food allergy'."[31] The skepticism comes from the fact that these doctors have had little experience with food allergy because it doesn't fit in with the immunological orientation, which is well understood. While the patient can sympathize with the doctors' desire to know what is going on, he is not willing to continue suffering from neglect just because theory can't explain why a method works. After all, aspirin has been used since the 19th century but only recently have researchers started to learn just how it functions in the body.

I am a sociologist, not a medical doctor, but what we are talking about here is as much sociological as medical, namely, how and why new ideas are adopted by a group or a society. Sociologists have long been concerned with the study of culture change and innovation, asking, for example, why the ancient Greeks did not put to practical use the steam engine which they invented and what kinds of farmers were the leaders in adopting hybrid seeds and new agricultural practices. Here we are concerned with the adoption by doctors of new medical concepts.

We tend to think of medicine as being highly progressive with doctors rushing to try the newest medicine or surgical technique as soon as it is developed. In many cases this is true, but not always with happy results. The new medicine may produce side effects which result in complications more serious than the original disease. Many patients fared poorly as their doctors rushed to try open heart surgery without adequate preparation.

In a number of ways though, medicine is very conservative. In the 19th century English doctors delayed for decades in adopting the stethoscope. Semmelweis concluded that the major cause of childbed fever in Europe was that the doctors were not washing their hands between examinations of patients. Despite his position as chief of the medical maternity division of Vienna General Hospital, he was unable to get his view accepted and finally died in an insane asylum, his mind broken by the thought of all the lives needlessly lost through refusal of the doctors to change.

More recently, Sister Elizabeth Kenny, an Australian nurse who developed a method for treating polio that reduced paralysis and limb deformation, battled half a lifetime just to get doctors to try her approach. Finally, some physicians in Minneapolis agreed to try her method and found it superior to the treatments which had been used. By the time it was generally accepted, the vaccine for polio had been developed, but a whole generation of people, many of them children, were deprived of the benefits of her discovery.

Allergy seems not to be different, its pioneers encountering rejection by the medical establishment. Dr. Arthur Coca was certainly a distinguished physician. He was Medical Director of Lederle Laboratories for 17 years, founder and first editor of the *Journal of Immunology*, and taught at three major universities. In the 1930's he discovered that the pulse of a person who is allergic to a substance will rise after exposure to that substance. He developed a system (which we shall look at later) for detecting allergies by monitoring the pulse and found that it made possible the alleviation of a wide variety of symptoms.

While not infallible, his system was a major advance, especially given the primitive state of development of allergy practice at the time. His first book, describing his method and some of the results he had obtained using it, was published in 1942. It was met with great resistance from the medical profession, so much so that he commented specifically on this in the 1945 second edition.

In the preface to this book, he complained of the hostile reception to his earlier edition by "experienced allergists and other medical specialists, from whom I could reasonably expect at least an unprejudiced hearing, if not generous cooperation." He continued: "The attitude of most of these towards the first edition of this monograph has been that of a skepticism so uncompromising that I have not even been invited to demonstrate the new method of examination described therein."[32] Note that it was not that other doctors tried his method and found it didn't work, but that they even refused to inform themselves about it.

Not only that, but without investigating his methods and results they told him to withdraw some of his claims. Coca wrote: "As to other symptoms that I have listed as food-allergic, I have been expressly advised by some allergists not to 'claim' a food-allergic etiology for these." One allergist friend of Coca's wrote expressing "fear and worry" over Coca's classification, "particularly since most of us are trying to prevent the term Allergy from being applied to anything and everything...."[33]

Again, it was not a matter of whether Coca was factually correct or not, but that he should not say what he had learned from his own experience because this contradicted established orthodoxy. One is reminded of Galileo having to deny before the Inquisition what his own observations told him was correct. Coca apparently gave up on trying to convince the medical profession and in 1956 wrote a book for laymen, *The Pulse Test,* which is still in print.

In 1951 three highly qualified allergists with backgrounds in both private practice and medical college teaching published a book, *Food Allergy,* which should have had a profound effect on the practice of allergy. It may yet. These men were Herbert J. Rinkel, Theron G. Randolph, and Michael Zeller. Like Coca they developed a new method of testing for allergies and found that they could alleviate a wide variety of symptoms by having the patient avoid foods which were allergenic for him. The book was generally received with a dull thud of silence.

They may have anticipated this on the basis of their earlier experience. They wrote: "There has been difficulty on the part of both physicians and patients to place existing knowledge into actual practice. As in the past, the ease to disbelieve a new concept frequently overcomes scientific curiosity and its attendent desires to explore a new field."[34]

Eleven years later Randolph published a landmark book, *Human Ecology and Susceptibility to the Chemical Environment,* which was a comprehensive treatment of allergy to chemical substances and air pollutants, thus anticipating by almost a decade scientific and popular interest in the environment. The book also has been very slow in getting recognition.

In 1976 Lawrence Dickey, a clinical ecologist, decried the failure of doctors even to investigate food allergy, saying that "food factors in disease, especially those of an allergic nature, are of great significance to those who have taken the trouble to become acquainted with the concepts and techniques of those who have devoted a great deal of time and energy to developing them. Unfortunately, this knowledge is not taught in medical school." He also charged that medical school allergists, who are immunologically oriented, "Have made no significant changes in either testing or specific antigen therapy since Noon and Freeman described them in 1911.[35]

Why this conservatism, this resistance to something new, particularly by people who are committed both to a scientific orientation relying on evidence to reveal the truth and to a humanistic concern with aiding the patient as much as possible through medical treatment? This is a sociological problem which I may investigate more fully some time in the future.

There are many facets to this issue but I will suggest one here. As noted earlier, the practice of allergy developed using skin tests for detecting allergens and giving shots to build up resistance to them, all within a secure scientific framework of immunology. Methods like Coca's and Rinkel-Randolph-Zeller's put the doctor in a theoretical no-man's-land and also involve the patient actively in the process of detecting allergens and make him more than just a needle recipient. These methods would drastically change the nature of the allergist's work, but the doctors who went into the field of allergy did so because they liked it the way it was. Change would not be welcome to them, hence they resist it. But the desire of conventional allergists to live in the simple world of the needle is not justification enough for depriving patients of the full benefits of modern medical knowledge.

We must recognize of course, though, that there are many conventional allergists practicing who have exerted themselves mightily for the benefit of their patients. They have visited homes and places of work and spent large quantities of time working with patients in order to ferret out the causes of their patients' troubles using the investigative genius of a Sherlock Holmes. Even conventional methods of food allergy detection can be quite effective if combined with a drive to really uncover the guilty substances. Once the culprits were located they spent more time advising patients on how to minimize the problems caused by allergy. I am sure the patients who have had such allergists are deeply grateful for their ability, efforts and devotion.

If allergists are not taught all of the concepts and methods that have been introduced into the field, imagine the amount of training given the average doctor. Writing in the 1960s, Jack and Burton Rudolph said: "The allergies have been neglected because the teaching of allergy is inadequate in most medical schools. The graduates of these schools are deficient in their understanding of allergic diseases, and therefore fail to recognize and treat them properly."[36] They noted that most medical men were not interested in allergy and did not want to specialize in the field.

Ten years later the situation was no different. The Rudolphs continued the above statement in a newer edition of their book and textbook author Lawrence Dickey wrote: "To most physicians, food allergy is well within the realm of fantasy.... The subject is not taught in medical schools. The immunologically oriented allergist does not consider it within his field of study...."[37] He went on to note that "The physician who stresses nutrition and food factors in disease is often looked upon as a food faddist." To get such a reputation is to suffer a great loss of status from the standpoint of the medical profession.

Finally, though, clinical ecology and its concepts are starting to attract attention both among doctors and the public. There have been a number of articles about allergy in lay publications, and books written from the clinical ecology point of view are starting to come out. Even the prestigious medical journal, *The Lancet,* had a favorable article concerning food allergy.[38] The writers of the latter, two Liverpool, England doctors, even felt it necessary to use quotation marks around the term, food allergy, for reasons which should be evident to the readers of this chapter.

They reported on six patients ranging from a 13-year-old girl to a 44-year-old man who collectively had symptoms including chest pains, heart palpitations, shortness of breath, depression, neurotic fears, throbbing headaches, slurred speech, back pains, vaginal ulcers, school behavior problems, abdominal pains, nausea and vomiting, sweating, fainting, and a general feeling of panic In attempts to diagnose or treat these individuals, doctors had used a variety of types of drugs and such medical procedures as skull X-ray, electroencephalogram (brain wave test), brainscan, angiogram, pyelogram, surgery, and even hypnotic sessions. In each case the symptoms were cleared up by detecting foods to which the patients were sensitive—tea, coffee, potato, tomato, and chocolate. The information in this article was ho-hum routine to Dr.

Theron Randolph 30 years earlier.

To make sure that the symptoms were caused by food and not the patients' expectations, the doctors in some cases administered substances through a tube directly to the stomach with the patient not knowing what was being given. The doctors concluded: "This clinical study supports the view that some foods may cause widespread and disabling symptoms in people who are sensitive to them."[39] Their explanation is simple and should be obvious to everyone, making it all the more strange that doctors generally have still not accepted it. "Since many diseases are caused by the interaction of man with the environment, and since one of the major environmental factors is food, it seems feasible that dietary factors may cause disease...."[40] This view is basic to clinical ecology.

These two English doctors imply that food allergy should be considered only for the "hard core" patients who are difficult or impossible to diagnose or treat with other means. I would suggest that, quite to the contrary, food allergy should be one of the first things to be considered. One reason is that it is so easy and quick to determine if food allergy is a factor in a particular case. While it may take some effort to track down particular trouble-causing foods, a few days of fasting or eating different foods (as described in chapter five) can show if food allergy in general is a cause of a particular symptom. Keeping in mind a few cautions to be mentioned later, it also is very safe. In contrast, the patients reported on in this article "underwent numerous investigations and treatments, some of which were potentially dangerous."[41]

We can hope that the *Lancet* article is just the first of many publications which will swing the medical profession around to a realization of the importance of environmental substances which can affect health. It is quite possible that even though clinical ecology has largely gone unrecognized for decades, it could quickly become an important force in medicine, one which would produce profound benefits for many patients.

We have seen, then, the explanation for the situation we started with, why despite the fact that allergy is so common it so frequently goes unrecognized. The result is that many people who could be helped remain untreated because of medical conservatism. I know; I was one of them. Behind many cases of both doctors and laymen who became interested in particular illnesses is a story of being affected by that condition and wanting to do something about it. My symptoms were respiratory. For other allergy sufferers they could be any of the conditions mentioned earlier or yet others. The only way to find out is to check for allergies. We will go into that later.

References

1. Vaughan, Warren T., M.D., *Allergy and Applied Immunology,* 2nd edit., C.V. Mosby Co., St. Louis, 1934, pp. 58-60.

2. Rudolph, Jack A., M.D., and Rudolph, Burton M., M.D., *Allergies: What They Are and What to do About Them,* Pyramid Books, New York, 1973, p. 15.

3. Hirschfeld, Herman, M.D., F.A.C.A., *The Whole Truth About Allergy,* Arco Publishing Co., New York, 1963, pp. 160-61.

4. Randolph, Theron G., M.D., "Historical Development of Clinical Ecology," in Dickey, Lawrence D., M.D. F.A.C.S., *Clinical Ecology,* Charles C. Thomas, Springfield, Ill., 1976, pp. 10-12.

5. Philpott, William H., M.D., "Maladaptive Reactions to Frequently Used Foods and Commonly Met Chemicals as Precipitating Factors in Many Chronic Physical and Chronic Emotional Illnesses," in Williams,

Roger J., Ph.D., and Kalita, Dwight K., Ph.D., *A Physician's Handbook on Orthomolecular Medicine,* Pergamon Press, New York, 1977, p. 140.

6. Rudolph and Rudolph, op. cit., p. 27.

7. Mackarness, Richard, M.D., *Eating Dangerously,* Harcourt, Brace, Jovanovich, New York, 1976, p. 26.

8. Coca, Arthur F., M.D., *The Pulse Test,* ARC Books, New York, 1959, p. 16.

9. Mandell, Marshall, M.D., "Cerebral Reactions in Allergic Patients: Illustrative Case Histories and Comments," in Williams and Kalita, op. cit., p. 136.

10. Challem, Jack Joseph, "An Exclusive Interview with 'The Children's Doctor,' Lendon H. Smith, M.D.," *Bestways,* August 1977, Vol 5, No. 8, pp. 17 and 18.

11. Coca, op. cit., p. 150.

12. Coca, Arthur F., M.D., *Familial Nonreaginic Food-Allergy,* 2nd edit., Charles C. Thomas, Springfield, Ill., 1945, pp. 68-69.

13. Sheldon, John M., M.D., Lovell, Robert G., M.D., and Mathews, Kenneth P., M.D., *A Manual of Clinical Allergy,* 2nd edit., W. D. Saunders Co., Philadelphia, 1967, pp. 196 and 200.

14. ibid., p. 200.

15. Hirschfeld, op. cit., p. 13.

16. Sherman, op. cit., p. 158.

17. Rinkel, Randolph, and Zeller, op. cit., p. 76.

18. ibid., p. 59.

19. Mandell, op. cit. and "Central Nervous System Hypersensitivity to House Dust, Molds, and Foods," in *Review of Allergy,* Vol 24, No. 4, pp. 293-94.

20. Sheldon, Lovell, and Mathews, op. cit., p. 200.

21. Mackarness, op. cit., p. 122.

22. ibid., p. 123.

23. Rinkel, Randolph, and Zeller, op. cit., pp. 357 and 104.

24. ibid., p. 104.

25. Feingold, Ben F., M.D., *Introduction to Clinical Allergy,* Charles C. Thomas, Springfield, Ill., 1973, p. 3.

26. Randolph, op. cit., p. 11.

27. Sherman, op. cit., p. 6.

28. ibid., p. 156.

29. Feingold, op. cit., p. 147.

30. Sherman, op. cit., p. 155.

31. ibid., p. 155.

32. Coca, *Familial Nonreaginic Food-Allergy,* p. vii.

33. ibid., p. 68.

34. Rinkel, Randolph, and Zoller, op. cit., p. 4.

35. Dickey, Lawrence D., M.D., F.A.C.S., *Clinical Ecology,* Charles C. Thomas, Springfield, Ill., 1976, pp. 33-34 and 5.

36. Rudolph, Jack A. and Rudolph, Burton M., *Victory Over Allergies,* Groton Press, New York, 1966, p. xi.

37. Dickey, op. cit., p. 26.

38. Finn, Ronald and Cohen, H. Newman, "'Food Allergy': Fact or Fiction?", *The Lancet,* Feb. 25, 1978, pp. 426-8.

39. ibid., p. 426.

40. ibid.

41. ibid., p. 427.

CHAPTER 2

My Personal Experience With Allergy

THE YEAR WAS 1940 and I was a teenager who had come to see a specialist in eye, ear, nose and throat conditions. He certainly seemed like an appropriate doctor to consult. I had frequent colds and recurrent earaches and an almost constant generous production of nasal mucus which was at its worst mornings and evenings. Getting to sleep at night was a battle between trying to breathe, blowing my nose, and the need for rest. Eventually fatigue would conquer the misery, but only for the moment. The next morning would find heavy mucus accumulation from during the night, which would require much nose blowing after arising. As I would blow I would hear noises in my ear. I knew about the Eustachian tube which connects the ears to the throat and that infections can travel up this tube. I was worried about deafness resulting from all this, but the need to breathe does not permit luxuries such as trying to preserve one's hearing.

The man probably would have been considered a "good doctor" both by other physicians and by laymen. Some relatives of mine thought highly of him, and he had his office in Minneapolis' most prestigeous location for doctors—the then-new downtown 20-story Medical Arts Building. Conversation was minimal. He led me into an examining room, looked in my nose, mouth and ears, took two long cotton-tipped sticks and inserted one way up into each nostril and walked out. Mucus flowed out copiously, which with the irritation of the swabs produced violent sneezing. There was a box of tissues handy but any attempt to use them jarred the swabs which increased both the mucus and the sneezing. He had said nothing about how long this treatment would go on. Five minutes? All afternoon? Would it help?

So there I sat, sneezing and wiping and wondering until he eventually returned and removed those spears pointed at my brain. If he made a diagnosis I never found out what it was. I do not recall any improvement resulting from his ministrations and never saw him again. As I sat in his examining room thinking that the procedure would be an excellent means of torture, neither I nor apparently the doctor realized that the treatment which I needed then had already been developed and reported in the medical literature.[1] Another 36 years was to go by before I learned of it and many doctors still haven't.

One day not long after my ordeal, I was in a downtown store and had my attention captured by a man demonstrating a preparation which seemed heaven-sent for my condition. I rapturously pictured the idyllic condition he described—of being able to breathe freely and easily, of going to bed and waking up without a feeling of suffocating. All it took was buying a bottle of his preparation and mixing a spoonful of it into a jar of melted petroleum jelly. The resulting concoction, rather similar to Vick's Vaporub, was to be applied in the nostrils in the evening. The very existence of the product and the fact a man could support himself selling it indicated that many others must have had similar problems.

I eagerly bought a bottle and rushed home to prepare the mixture that would enable me to enter the easy-breathing Nirvana that I could envision so clearly. The active ingredients, guessed at from a hazy recollection, were probably menthol, camphor, and the like. I wound up making several batches of the stuff and using it for some time. It really didn't help that much but at least I felt I was doing something.

Whether from maturation or a change of environment and diet, occasioned by entering the army during World War II, I improved and remained so after marriage and returning to civilian life. But eventually many of the old symptoms returned, so 25 years after my original encounter with a nose and throat specialist I consulted another one. After all, a quarter of a century had elapsed and medical research had attained heights of accomplishment that were undreamed of before—the "wonder drugs," open heart surgery, a vaccine for polio, new laboratory diagnostic tests, sophisticated new machines such as artificial hearts and kidneys, electronic heart pacemakers, and on and on. Surely something would have been developed for my stuffy nose and recurrent colds and flu.

After a brief examination the doctor gave me his diagnosis—chronic rhinitis. Chronic means regular or recurrent and rhinitis is the medical term for inflamation of the mucous membranes of the nose. All he did was to express in medical terminology what I already knew. But what could be done? Now he would certainly give me one of those miraculous new medical discoveries that would solve my problem. What he did do was prescribe an antihistamine-decongestant tablet. While this helped with the day-to-day stuffiness it did not do anything to reduce the frequent bouts with cold and flu, and after a couple of years I came down with such a severe case of pneumonia that it took a whole year to fully recover.

Hardly was I over that when I became aware of something physically wrong in the nose-throat area. Consulting yet a third nose and throat specialist revealed that I had developed nasal polyps, benign sac-like growths or enlargements of the mucous tissues, which needed to be removed surgically. The operation is not a major one; I was able to go home the next day and was largely back to normal within a week. The polyps left their mark though. They had blocked off nasal passages and sinuses, and a resulting infection produced an almost complete permanent loss of the sense of smell. During the follow-up examination the doctor remarked almost incidentally that polyps frequently result from allergies and suggested seeing an allergist.

The one I consulted was the ideal age for a doctor, somewhere around 40, young enough to have had a recent medical education but old enough to have acquired the depth of knowledge that comes from experience. He gave me skin tests for 40 different substances and informed me that I was allergic to housedust, mold and weeds. The treatment would be a series of shots, three a week at first but tapering off to one a week and continuing for five years. The shots would contain the materials I was allergic to and were intended to increase my resistance to those substances. This is a standard treatment for allergies.

The three allergens discovered did not include any foods. I learned later that skin tests are very unreliable for foods. The doctor did mention one food as a frequent trouble-causer—milk. He suggested I could test this by going two or three days without any and see if I felt better. You will see later why this advice was exactly the opposite of the proper way to test for food sensitivity. He also gave me an antihistamine-decongestant prescription which I found it necessary to use regularly.

Each shot made my arm sore for four or five days afterward so the doctor suggested trying half the dose in each arm. This resulted in two sore arms per time so I went back to the original system. For three years straight I had at least one almost continuously sore arm. Of course it would have been worth it had there been a marked improvement, but this was not the case and what there was probably owed more to the decongestant than the shots. I still consumed boxes of tissues at an alarming rate.

After three years of this I came down with yet another cold, but one which led to pneumonia and asthma. For months I would be awakened in the middle of the night by the sound of my own wheezing. In desperation, while shopping one day, my wife picked up a copy of Adelle Davis' *Let's Get Well,* hoping that somewhere in those pages we would find something helpful. I, who had never been interested in learning about medical things, became fascinated by the existence of the vast body of medical and health literature which Adelle Davis referred to and started reading voraciously on these subjects.

Davis emphasized the B-vitamin pantothenic acid for allergies so I started taking this. I had already been taking vitamin C. Further reading led to taking additional vitamin supplements and altering our diet to replace junk foods with more nutritious natural foods. The changes produced an incredible increase in energy and vigor in my wife and produced measurable benefits for me. Within a few months I lost 20 unneeded pounds. My blood pressure, which was right on the borderline of being considered high, 150/100, dropped to a normal 120/80. About the time we started making these dietary changes I had been shocked to learn that my blood cholesterol and, more even serious, my blood triglycerides were quite high, 336 and 364 respectively. While the cholesterol remained around 300 the triglycerides dropped to 124. (At my most recent check, after having gotten my allergies under control, cholesterol was 230 and triglycerides 110).

While it was gratifying to know that lowered readings indicated a substantially lesser risk of heart attack, and I felt better generally and exceptional some days, I still had the frequent cold and nasal symptoms. In my reading I came across Coca's *The Pulse Test*, which tells how to test for allergies by taking one's pulse (more of this later) and tested carefully for the foods I was eating but could not detect anything definite.

So there I was. I had tried all that medical science and the health movement had to offer and I still had most of the problems I had had earlier. I was on a regular cycle of two to three weeks in which I would have a "cold" and then get better only to repeat the process again and again. I would catch a cold in December and be unable to breathe through my nose during most of January and sometimes into February. I would buy boxes of tissues a half a dozen at a time and replenish my bedside container and fill the wastebasket beside my living room chair at an astonishing rate. All of a sudden my nose would start running or I would start sneezing for no apparent reason. Although I learned later that it could all be explained, at the time it was all an unfathomable mystery.

Then the Ohio chapter of the Huxley Institute for Biosocial Research held a conference at nearby Bowling Green State University. The Institute, with its national headquarters in New York City, is primarily an information and referral center concerned with encouraging the use and spread of orthomolecular medicine. This term, which was introduced by the distinguished scientist Linus Pauling in 1968, refers to the treatment of medical conditions with "right molecules" (which is what orthomolecular means).

Such treatment emphasizes diet, vitamins and minerals in preference to drugs, although more conventional medicines and treatments may be used by orthomolecular physicians if necessary. Clinical ecology as described in the preceding chapter would be considered as part of orthomolecular medicine, as it examines man's environment for evidence of factors that can affect health or produce illness in susceptible individuals. It emphasizes identifying and minimizing the effect of environmental exposures rather than using drugs to cover up symptoms or alter the body processes.[2]

In psychiatry, the orthomolecular approach earlier was called mega-vitamin treatment and was pioneered by psychiatrists Abram Hoffer and Humphrey Osmond, who found that massive doses of certain vitamins were helpful in treating schizophrenia. Because of this background the Institute's program is oriented heavily toward psychiatry, which is very evident from the fact that its Canadian affiliate is called the Canadian Schizophrenia Foundation. Nevertheless, the Institute's interests go beyond psychiatry to include any branch of medicine where orthomolecular concepts are appropriate. Also, orthomolecular psychiatrists have been drawn into the field of allergy as they have come to realize that, for some people, allergy results not in a runny nose or a skin rash but rather in abnormal behavior.

Although I got valuable information from the Bowling Green conference itself, both from the presentations and from literature which was available there, my interest was aroused to the point that I wanted to find out still more about allergy in general and clinical ecology in particular. I took advantage of the medical college library here in Toledo to do additional reading. All of this finally gave me the knowledge that I had needed for so many years.

While I would rather have used the services of a clinical ecologist, there are none in town so I decided to go ahead on my own. Using methods which I shall later describe I was able within a few weeks to determine that I had sensitivities to a number of foods I had been eating regularly. I have since found additional foods to which I am allergic, and would probably be considered a rather severe case of food allergy.

How can a person regularly eat foods without realizing he is allergic to them? This is what clinical ecology explains so well. By learning which foods were causing trouble for me and avoiding them I was able to break my cycle of illnesses. I felt I must pass this information on. Hence this book.

References

1. Elimination diets, (to be described later) had been developed and reported on in the 1920's. They were discussed, among other places, in Vaughan, Warren T., M.D., *Allergy and Applied Immunology,* 2nd edit., C. V. Mosby Co., St. Louis, 1934, in Vaughan's 1939 *Practice of Allergy,* C. V. Mosby, and in Rowe, Albert H., M.D., *Food, Inhalant and Other Clinical Allergy,* Lea and Febiger, Philadelphia, 1937. Even though not ideal, I am sure elimination diets would have been successful in detecting the milk and cereal grains to which I am sensitive.

2. See Randolph, Theron G., M.D., "Historical Development of Clinical Ecology," in Dickey, Lawrence D., M.D., F.A.C.S., *Clinical Ecology,* Charles C. Thomas, Springfield, Ill., 1976, pp. 10–12.

CHAPTER 3

The Wacky World
of Allergy

ALLERGY IS A condition in which the body reacts in some way to a substance which produces some reaction in the body, that substance being one which does not produce such a reaction in the majority of people. This definition is very broad, but necessarily so because both the kinds of substances and the kinds of reactions are so varied. Any substance which produces an allergic reaction is called an allergen. The adjective allergenic is used to describe such a substance.

While some substances produce allergic reactions more commonly than others, when a substance is referred to as allergenic it is always with regard to the reactions of certain people. In other words, allergy is a matter of some people's sensitivities to a substance, not to any characteristic inherent in the material itself. The words sensitivity and allergy may be considered interchangeable in this context.

There are several ways in which allergens can reach the body: (1) as foods or medicines which are ingested, (2) as inhalants, either as minute solids (dusts, pollen, etc.) or as gases or liquid droplets in the air being breathed, (3) as materials which come into contact with the surface of the body, such as clothing, externally applied medications or cosmetics, or anything handled or contacted in some way by the skin, or (4) as additives to or contaminants of the above three. Number (4) emphasizes that a person might not be sensitive to a food itself but to an additive or pesticide or preservative that had been applied to the food. Similarly, a person might be susceptible to chemicals in drinking water, or to the permanent press finish used on cloth rather than to the material itself. We are indebted to Dr. Theron Randolph for his emphasis on chemical contaminants.

Some substances may reach the body in more than one way. Wheat, for example, most commonly is a food allergen, but, for people such as bakers exposed to flour dust in food preparation, it is an inhalant. A person may be allergic to the material in its inhalant form but not as a food, or vice versa, or to both forms. In the latter case, the symptoms may be different for the different forms—asthma from inhaling and hives from eating, for example.[1] Allergists are very aware of flax, which may be a food, an inhalant (it is widely used industrially), and a contact allergen in the form of linen.

There is widespread agreement that allergies tend to run in families. A person who has two allergic parents has a greater chance of developing allergy than someone with only one allergic parent. The chances for allergy decrease as the number and closeness of relationship decrease. Estimates by different allergists have been in the range of 65% to 75% of allergy for children of two allergic parents, and 35% to 50% where only one parent is allergic.[2]

Considering the amount of undetected allergy, however, particularly for older generations, it is quite likely that if all cases of allergy were recognized the percentages would be higher. In my own case, for example, I was 45 years old and had consulted a number of doctors before one suggested I had allergies. What is transmitted hereditarily is a general tendency toward allergy, not a specific sensitivity or pattern of reaction. The parent may be sensitive to one substance, the child to another, and each can show different symptoms. In one instance the mother had intestinal systems while her son had hay fever.[3]

Allergies may be highly specific, as when a person reacts to Siamese but not to Persian cats, or to collie but not terrier dogs.[4] One man could eat Maine potatoes but not those from Rhode Island.[5] In this case it was not the potato itself to which he was sensitive but the particular molds naturally associated with foods that were specific to the Rhode Island soil. Differences in molds will also be responsible for a person reacting to one kind of spring water but not to another. Also, some allergic reactions may be confined to only one side of the body.[6]

Conventional allergy practice has been most successful with the hayfever type of inhalant allergies and with contact allergies. It has been much less so with food allergies for reasons that will be gone into as we go along. The main concern in this book is with food allergies and their detection.

Given the complex slippery nature of allergy, it is a wonder that its characteristics could ever be tracked down. Yet, because this would not have required any of our modern technology, it could have been done thousands of years ago. Indeed, Hippocrates made some astute observations some 2,400 years ago which if followed up could have led to breakthroughs in ancient times.

The average person trying to make sense out of his symptoms faces a maze of problems and apparent contradictions. Are these symptoms caused by allergy? Maybe its because something else is wrong with me. But the doctors tell me they can't find anything wrong; all my tests are normal. Could it be wheat? No, I've always eaten bread and cereal and I didn't used to have these problems. How about milk? No, I tried going without that for awhile and I felt worse than ever. Could it be eggs? No, I always feel better after I eat them. Could it be tuna? I felt worse after supper last night when we had tuna. No, because it didn't bother me when I had tuna last week. And so it goes. Owing heavily to the work of Herbert Rinkel and Theron Randolph we are now able (and have been since 1951) to find our way through this bramble patch of uncertainties. In their book, *Food Allergy,* Rinkel, Randolph and Zeller (to be referred to hereafter as RRZ) give a clear picture of how allergy works and tell how to test accurately and specifically for food allergies. Let us take a look at the picture of allergy which they present.

First, allergies may be either "fixed" or "cyclic". Fixed allergies are those, in effect, the person is born with and are permanent. Some infants show allergy to a food the first time they are exposed to it; there is no question of having become allergic to it through long and repeated exposure. No matter how long you avoid a fixed allergen you will still be sensitive to it.

Cyclic allergies are those you are not born with but develop as a result of repeated exposure to a food. The amount of exposure required to sensitize a person varies greatly from one person to another. Because a person is not born with the sensitivity to an allergen which is cyclic for him he can usually lose the sensitivity by avoiding that food for a length of time. In other words, he can revert to a state where he is no longer sensitive to the food. Then, by not eating it too often he can include it in his diet without it causing trouble.

How long a period of time is required to lose the sensitivity and how often one can later eat the food with impunity is highly variable for different people. In general, one should avoid the food for three months and then test for sensitivity (the test method will be described later). If still sensitive, then repeat another three month cycle of avoidance and then test again. RRZ are not ready to call an allergy fixed unless one is still sensitive after two years of such cycles.

Some people may lose their sensitivity to a food within two or three weeks. If you are really curious about a food you can test for sensitivity sooner than three months. But it may be that having dropped the food from your diet you learn to live without it and have no strong desire for it. Of course there is no reason why you should go back to eating it except that from the standpoint of your overall nutrition you want to see that you get an adequate diet. This last point is quite important because allergic people might wind up eating a rather limited selection of foods.

Once having lost sensitivity to a food a person can reacquire it by eating the food too frequently. Only experience will show what degree of frequency is too much for a particular person. One can start with once a week and if no problems result then can try twice a week. A few people may be able to tolerate a greater frequency—every other day, or possibly every day. A person may find that once a day is OK but twice a day causes a reaction. Frequency of eating is more important in determining reactions than the amount eaten at any one time.

Of course any time a person gets resensitized to a food another period of avoidance will be needed. When the sensitivity has been lost again then one should try eating the food at only half the frequency at which sensitivity was reacquired. That is, if the person got an allergic reaction eating the food twice a week then he should not eat it oftener than once a week.

Are some foods more allergenic than others? Undoubtedly, but frequency of use of a food also seems to be very important. There is considerable agreement in the literature that the foods most frequently found to be allergenic are milk, eggs, wheat and corn. One recent book lists the most common food allergens as given by nine different authors. Milk is clearly number one. Dr. Frederic Speer's list is least typical with chocolate ranking second and much higher than wheat, but Speer specializes in children's allergies.[7]

It seems quite clear that the most common food allergens are precisely those which are most widely eaten. Potato, orange, beef and pork are also repeatedly mentioned, but these are common foods too. If everyone ate kumquats every day they too would probably be high on the list of allergens.

There appear to be geographic and cultural differences in the incidence of particular foods as allergens. Although rice is mentioned by some writers as being an infrequent allergen, this is probably because it is less commonly eaten than wheat or corn. RRZ found that wheat-sensitive patients who had eaten rice infrequently were not allergic to it, but that those who had eaten it frequently did show a reaction to it.[8]

There is the possibility that foods which are closely related to each other can each affect an individual in about the same way. Wheat, rye, and barley are similar genetically, for example, and a high proportion of people who are sensitive to one also react to the other two. There is a considerable amount of cross-sensitivity to the whole cereal grass family, which in addition to the above mentioned three also includes corn, millet, oats, rice, and sugar cane. Cross-sensitivities are also likely with members of the legume family—beans (including soybeans), lentils, peas and peanuts. Buckwheat, despite its name, is not a cereal grass but rather is a relative of rhubarb. Even if one is tolerant of buckwheat, it should not be eaten too often because as RRZ comment, "experience has taught us that most people become allergic to it when used regularly."[9]

According to the rotation diet principles described in Chapter 9, this would mean not oftener than once in four days. That same chapter also has tables of food family classifications.

Taking food family relationships into account means that finding a sensitivity to one member of the family suggests that one should check to see if there is a reaction to other members of that family. It can also mean that a person has a greater likelihood of becoming allergic to a presently innocent food which is related to one to which the person is sensitive. In my own case, in the process of avoiding wheat I ate millet fairly regularly and developed a reaction to that. Despite the similarity of wheat and rye I have a greater tolerance for rye than for wheat. Thus, while biological classification of foods may offer some clues, each food still needs to be considered in its own right.

Studies of the extent to which particular foods are found to be allergenic in a large population are of interest to the medical researcher but only of marginal value to the individual. For the person trying to determine which foods, if any, he is allergic to it doesn't help a great deal to know that 20% of the people who were studied by Doctor X were allergic to food Y. The question the person needs to have answered is, to what foods am I sensitive?

What this amounts to is that the answer to allergy is not to be found in the characteristics of foods, but in those of the person who is eating them. About all one can say is that if a person is having chronic troubles from food allergy, the guilty foods have to be among those that are eaten regularly. So we need to refocus our attention on the allergic person.

There are other complicating factors influencing food allergy which were pointed out by RRZ. Some people show "concomitant" sensitivity. Such people are only sensitive to a food when they are also being subjected to an inhalant which affects them, such as pollen or dust. In addition to it being unfair, in that the person is only hit by it when he is already under attack from another enemy, it also may complicate the task of detecting the guilty food.

People sensitive to house dust are affected most in the winter when they are cooped up in a closed house. The hay fever victim might acquire food allergies when his hay fever is active in the late summer. About the only way concomitant sensitivity would be revealed would be if the person found that he was sensitive to a food at one time but not another. Another implication of concomitant allergy is that a person might be sensitive to a food in one part of the country where he is exposed to certain inhalant allergens but not in another region where the plant pollens or chemicals in the air are different.

One might be allergic to a food when cooked but not when raw or vice versa. Likewise a fresh fruit might be allergenic for a person but not the dried form. Nevertheless, if a person finds he can tolerate one form of a food but not another he should still be cautious about frequency of eating it so that the sensitivity does not spread to all forms of the food.

A person sensitive to a whole food may or may not react to a substance which represents only a fraction of that food. A person allergic to beets, for example, may also be susceptible to beet sugar, and one who reacts to corn may also be affected by corn syrup or corn oil.

A relatively small number of people have "thermal" sensitivity to foods. They will get a reaction to the consumption of a food only if it is followed by exposure to heat or cold. RRZ recommend that such people try to increase their tolerance by exposing themselves to temperatures which they find somewhat uncomfortable. A person sensitive to cold, for example, who wears heavy clothing and keeps the room temperature high will reduce his tolerance as time goes by and become increasingly susceptible to cooler temperatures and their associated food allergy problems. As another means of combatting sensitivity to cold they recommend alternate hot and cold showers, each several minutes long, twice a day. Avoiding the foods which cause a reaction during the winter is also recommended.[10]

A few persons are light-sensitive, developing food allergies when they are exposed to much light as during the summer. If they keep themselves shaded or covered with clothing they do not have problems with foods.

Individuals vary a great deal in their sensitivity or "inherent tolerance." Those with low tolerance become sensitized easily or quickly. Individuals with high tolerance can eat foods long and frequently before becoming sensitized. The low tolerance person will generally be sensitive to half or more of the foods ordinarily eaten. Tolerance is not necessarily related to severity of symptoms. Thus, a high tolerance person may take much exposure before coming sensitive to a food but have a strong reaction when he finally is affected, or the opposite could be true. The person with the most severe problems would be the low tolerance person who shows severe symptoms.

The literature on allergy contains cases of people with such exquisite sensitivity that even the most minute contact with a food produced a reaction. Some people have been affected by a food just from being in the kitchen when it was being cooked. People extremely sensitive to milk have responded when eating chicken or veal that was milk-fed. A small number of people may be so sensitive to milk that they cannot tolerate beef. Individuals extremely sensitive to egg have been affected by eating female chickens, some of the hormones in a laying chicken being the same as those in the eggs. One woman has been reported who could tell at first bite whether a chicken was male or female.

If there is one food which can produce extreme reactions for those supersensitive to it in even the tiniest amounts it is egg. People sensitive to eggs have developed rashes just from handling the shells. One boy known to be allergic to egg had a special egg-free birthday cake made for him but a cake containing eggs was also made for the other children. The cake containing egg was cut first, the knife was then wiped off and then used to cut the egg-free cake. Just the miniscule amount of egg remaining on the knife was enough to make the boy sick.[11] Allergists are urged to be cautious even in doing skin tests for egg, although as Dr. Feingold has pointed out, an individual who is strongly sensitive to egg usually knows about it from experience.[12]

Even for people whose food sensitivities are more typical, trying to avoid certain foods in our complex world can be a real problem. The most common allergens, wheat, corn, milk, and eggs are also the most widespread. Randolph considers corn the leading allergen at present, the major difficulty being that it is used in so many different ways.[13] Avoiding whole corn—canned, frozen, or on the cob—is of course no problem but other forms may not be noticed unless one is very observant.

Feingold lists more than 150 products containing corn, many in an unsuspected and undetectable form.[14] Corn content may not always be shown on the label of a product if it has a label. Stamps and envelope adhesives may contain corn and while even the extra-sensitive person might not be affected by posting a note to Aunt Gertrude, stamping and sealing a batch of cards at holiday time might be another matter. Paper plates and cartons can have a corn product used in their manufacture which is picked up by food or beverage coming into contact with them. Aspirin tablets and other medications as well as vitamin tablets may contain corn. Corn may also show up in beer, liquor and even wine. It is an ingredient in some toothpastes. In foods it may be in peanut butter, pickles, and vinegar. In a more recognizable form it may appear as corn meal on breaded meat or fish. Both corn syrup and its related products, dextrose and glucose, and corn oil are widely used in food preparation. Some margarines contain corn oil. There are cases of people sensitive to corn who got a reaction from eating ham or bacon because of the corn syrup used in the curing process. Truly, the lot of the person who is highly sensitive to corn can be a difficult one.

Wheat also is very widespread and in its more common forms will certainly be recognized—bread and wheat cereal. Most gravies will contain wheat. Label reading will frequently reveal wheat as an ingredient in products which are identified according to other grains. Ready-to-eat oat cereal (Cheerios) has wheat in it as does almost all "rye" bread which is sold in supermarkets. Health food stores usually have wheat-free rye bread, although even this is relative. Because of the similarity of wheat and rye in growing and handling, some wheat is very likely to be mixed in with rye grain and flour.[15] For this reason alone a person highly sensitive to wheat is likely to react to rye. Wheat is also used in making meat-substitute products and may be an ingredient in sausage and luncheon meats.

Eggs and milk will easily be recognized in their primary forms but may show up in ways less obvious or expected. Dried powdered milk (nonfat milk solids) is included in many prepared foods. Most margarines contain milk solids although "diet" or "artificial" margarines usually do not. These, however, have other ingredients to which a person could be sensitive. There are brands of milk-free margarine sold in health food stores which are more natural. Nondairy coffee "creamers" may contain powdered milk. No-cholesterol egg substitutes contain egg white. Some people may be able to tolerate egg yolk but not the white. Some brands of commercial mayonnaise are made with whole eggs, other with just the yolk. Egg is frequently used as a binder in meat loafs.

When buying cans or packages of food at the supermarket certainly one should read the list of ingredients on the label. For some types of products, though, the government does not require that all ingredients be listed or that the substance be fully identified. Food additives may be a problem. Monosodium glutamate, or MSG, is a commonly used flavor enhancer in prepared foods and is not always listed on labels. It may be made from wheat, corn or sugar beets. If a food is made with shortening containing the preservative BHT, the label need only list the shortening. Even as simple a product as canned peas is likely to contain unlisted corn syrup.

The simplest solution to the problem, at least in the early stages of avoiding certain foods while testing, is to buy food raw as produce rather than packages of processed food. Read the list of ingredients on a box of instant mashed potatoes and you will know why you should buy potatoes raw and boil or bake them yourself. Similarly, prepared puddings, frozen pot pies and canned hash, stew and soups contain far too many ingredients to be sure of what one is or is not avoiding. Simple frozen fruits or vegetables will generally be uncontaminated with other ingredients, but of course an item like frozen peas in butter sauce should be passed by.

Allergens may be received in the course of medical treatments. Medicines themselves may be allergenic or they may be in a tablet or liquid which is allergenic. Vitamins, or more frequently, the fillers or binders used to make up the tablets may cause sensitivity in some people. In either case it may be possible to find another brand of the medicine or vitamin which is made up differently and does not cause trouble. Vaccines produced through the use of eggs can produce a reaction for egg-sensitive people. Glucose solutions administered intravenously, usually during hospitalization, could cause problems for corn-sensitive individuals. Anyone knowing of any allergic sensitivities who is getting medical treatment should be sure to inform the doctors and nurses of any known or suspected allergies.

Some people are sensitive to substances in ordinary water.[16] Chlorine, which is widely used by local water treatment plants to kill bacteria in water, may affect some people adversely. Fluorides in water may also cause reactions. Water which has been drawn from rivers or lakes is likely to contain a number of chemicals from industrial wastes and from run-off from agricultural land which has been subjected to pesticides, herbicides and fertilizers. Most water treatment plants are not equipped to detect and remove all these chemicals. The subject of chemicals as allergens is dealt with in a later chapter; only enough is being mentioned here to indicate the possible range of allergens and to give some understanding for allergy testing, also described later, because reactions to water could interfere with the interpretation of food tests.

Bottled spring water is ordinarily recommended for those sensitive to tap water, but this is not always completely simple. Even some underground water may have picked up contaminants, and different waters can have different natural molds to which some people will be sensitive. Bottled water may also be contaminated chemically during the bottling process, as from tubing or rubber gaskets the water comes in contact with, or from tap water used to wash out the bottles prior to filling them. Plastic bottles themselves may affect the water enough to produce a reaction in some people, so that glass bottles are preferable.

One may rid water of chlorine by letting it stand open for three days, by boiling it briefly, or by using an activated charcoal filter. The charcoal filter would also remove a number of other chemicals. Distilled water is a possibility, at least when one is making initial food tests, but it lacks minerals found in ordinary water that aid health and probably help to prevent heart attack. A person using distilled water on a long term basis should be sure of getting adequate mineral supplementation. More commonly, clinical ecologists have their patients try different brands of spring water until one is found that does not cause troubles for the person.

Although breast milk is not allergenic in itself, it can contain allergens if the mother has eaten something somewhat earlier to which the baby is sensitive.[17] Also, both children and adults can be affected by the penicillin which is frequently found in cow's milk as a residue from treatment of some cows for infections of the udder, etc.[18]

The other, and probably more common way, for the baby to be affected by cow's milk is when traces of it reach the baby through the mother's milk. Even if the mother herself seems not to be allergic to milk, enough of it may get through into her own milk to produce a reaction in a sensitive baby. Nursing mothers who drink milk generously for its calcium and other nutrients should be aware of this possibility. Other foods or spices could act similarly.

All of this should make it quite evident that people with allergies can find their lives are complicated by their condition, the extent of their difficulties being determined by the number, kind and degree of their sensitivities. It would be nice if the condition could be cured by just popping a few pills. Alas, it is not to be. While, as we shall see, there may be some possibilities for alleviating allergic reactions, avoidance of allergens is basic.

Serious cases may require major changes in living habits. Travel or eating away from home can produce symptoms from unexpected ingredients in food. Easy-to-fix prepared foods from the supermarket may be out as well as ones that have been favorite standbys in the diet for years. The person whose discomforts have been great enough will be willing to make the effort to locate the offenders and arrange things so as to minimize contact with them.

References

1. Rinkel, Herbert J., M.D., Randolph, Theron G., M.D. and Zeller, Michael, M.D., *Food Allergy,* Charles C. Thomas, Springfield, Ill. 1951, p. 67.

2. ibid., p. 55; Rudolph, Jack A., M.D., and Rudolph, Burton, M., M.D., *Allergies: What They Are and What to do About Them,* Pyramid Books, New York, 1973, p. 29; Kantor, Julius M., M.D., "Heredity of Allergy," in Speer, Frederic, M.D. and Dockhorn, Robert J., M.D., *Allergy and Immunology in Childhood,* Charles C. Thomas, Springfield, Ill., 1973, pp. 7–8.

3. Rinkel, Randolph, and Zeller, op. cit., p. 56.

4. Hirschfeld, Herman, M.D., F.A.C.A., *The Whole Truth About Allergy,* Arco Publishing Co., New York, 1963, p. 26.

5. Rinkel, Randolph, and Zeller, op. cit., p. 58.

6. Newbold, H. L., M.D., *Cerebral Allergic Reactions to Drinking Water,* presentation at Canadian Schizophrenia Foundation Annual Meeting, Windsor, Ontario, Canada, June 1977.

7. Speer and Dockhorn, op. cit., p. 397.

8. Rinkel, Randolph, and Zeller, op. cit., p. 256.

9. ibid., p. 237.

10. Rinkel, Randolph, and Zeller, op. cit., p. 84.

11. Newbold, H. L., op. cit.

12. Feingold, Ben F., M.D., *Introduction to Clinical Allergy,* Charles C. Thomas, Springfield, Ill., 1973, p. 151.

13. Challem, Jack Joseph, "An Exclusive Interview with Dr. Theron Randolph, M.D., *Bestways,* June 1977, p. 26.

14. Feingold, op. cit., p. 152.

15. Rinkel, Randolph, and Zeller, op. cit., p. 257.

16. see Morgan, Joseph T., M.D., "The Water Problem," in Dickey, Lawrence D., M.D., ed., *Clinical Ecology,* Charles C. Thomas, Springfield, Ill., 1976, pp. 306–309.

17. Feingold, op. cit., p. 151.

18. ibid., p. 163.

CHAPTER 4

Masking and Allergy-Addiction

IN ORDER TO be successful in detecting allergens, one must understand in practical terms how the body responds to them. This is no problem in the case of the person whose face breaks out in a rash two minutes after eating, say, strawberries. The outbreak follows immediately after eating the offending food and that person learns all he needs to know about strawberries—they are not for him. There is no difficulty in determining the source of such an instant reaction and so we will not be concerned with it here. Most people do not produce as clear cut symptoms as quickly as this, however, and can have real problems in trying to find the offenders.

We are indebted to Dr. Herbert J. Rinkel for the crucial insights that make the food allergy reaction process comprehensible. Rinkel is another example of a person whose interest in a medical question was stimulated by his own problem, for he too suffered from allergies. His ideas as they developed into an overall view of food allergy and were influenced by the work of others are presented in the 1951 book *Food Allergy,* written by Rinkel, Randolph and Zeller, a work which I have already mentioned. The ideas and methods described in that book represent a real breakthrough which as yet is not appreciated by most of the medical profession.

If you think you may have food allergies, before reading any more in this book take a sheet of paper and write out answers to the following questions:

1. Are there some foods to which you think you may be allergic? If so, what are they?

2. Are there some foods you eat at least two or three times a week that you are quite sure you are not allergic to? If so, what are they?

3. What are your favorite foods?

4. What foods do you consume at least once every day or two?

5. What foods regularly in your diet could you give up most easily if need be in order to control your allergies?

6. What foods would you most dislike having to give up if need be in order to control your allergies?

If you have food allergies it is almost certain that your main troublemakers are included in your answers to the above questions. Before we go on to methods for locating them we must see how allergy works.

The most important concept to get here is the idea of *masking*. This refers to the way the body may mask or cover up a response to a food it really is allergic to. The masking process is not greatly different whether the allergy is a permanent or a cyclic one. If a permanent one, let us say for milk, the baby will usually have troubles, probably digestive, when given a formula. Parents or doctor may recognize milk as guilty and substitute soybean milk which the baby tolerates well. But as the child grows up it keeps getting exposed to milk in baked goods, ice cream, etc. and the body gradually adapts to it.

Everyone says that the child has "outgrown" the allergy. True, there is no longer an acute reaction but the basic sensitivity to the food is no doubt still there. RRZ take issue with the "majority of texts" which claim allergy is more a childhood than an adult problem.[1] What has happened is that the sensitivity became masked by an adaptation of the body, but the adaptation itself creates stress and sooner or later is very likely to break down, resulting in illness of one type or another.

Another allergist, writing more recently, expresses a similar opinion: "Many fathers and mothers have the mistaken idea that children outgrow their allergies. They think the child is no longer allergic because the symptoms frequently disappear around the age of four or five years. Experience has proven this false. Careful studies show that the baby who reacts to eggs, milk or other allergens usually becomes the child or adult who suffers from other allergies in other ways.... Allergy is a versatile disease. Like a talented actor, it appears first as hives or eczema, then leaves and returns later as asthma or hay fever.[2]

As we shall see, allergy may also cause behavioral problems. I saw a case which illustrates these things while visiting as an observer the clinic operated by Dr. Marshall Mandell in Norwalk, Connecticut. A man in his thirties had a number of complaints including obsessive thoughts, and depression so serious that he had attempted suicide and had to be confined in a mental hospital for a number of months. When he was a boy he did not like tomato, but because the family was Italian his father made him eat tomato sauce on the pasta dishes which they had constantly, saying, "You're Italian, so you got to eat the pasta sauce." The boy got used to eating tomato and didn't think any more about it until Dr. Mandell's testing decades later revealed a sensitivity to tomato.

It is not uncommon for children to resist foods to which they are sensitive, but everyone tells them that this or that food is "good for them," or as in this case, that it is a matter of ethnic pride. So they get pressured into eating it regularly, adapt to it so that it appears to cease causing trouble, and it looks as though they have "outgrown" their sensitivity, only to have problems develop later.

For cyclic allergies the situation is not greatly different. The person eats a certain food every day or so. The body, which was able to tolerate it at first, gradually starts responding with symptoms of one kind or another, but the person does not recognize the relationship between the food and the symptoms, and so keeps eating the food. It is even likely to be one of his favorites. The symptoms or conditions which develop can include any one or more of the 100 which were listed in the first chapter.

This, then, is masking. A food which causes a physical reaction in one way or another appears innocent to the individual. There is no response that follows shortly after eating the food which indicates that it is guilty. The reaction goes underground and all the person knows is that he has headaches, digestive difficulties or whatever.

A food allergen which is masked will be undetectable to the affected person. As RRZ state: "Actually, the most discerning patient is rarely ever able to detect the presence of a masked food allergy. In fact, the most skilled allergist cannot do so either until he tests for it. Masking may be 100% perfect, even with an individual food test, if steps have not been taken to avoid it."[3] Let us see how the allergen may be unmasked.

The key to the unmasking process was discovered by Rinkel, out of his experience with his own allergies. Suffering from chronic runny nose, sore throats and ear infections he started experimenting with his own diet to see if foods could be causing his troubles. He had eaten eggs every day for years but found he felt better within a few days after eliminating them from his diet. However, after going without eggs for five days he ate a piece of cake without realizing that it contained egg. Ten minutes later he fainted. Analyzing his reaction afterward led him to conclude that the period of going without eggs had decreased his tolerance for them, giving him a quick response to the food.[4]

Fortunately, most people consuming an allergenic food after a period of avoidance do not get as drastic a reaction as did Rinkel and he developed a system for testing foods through avoidance and re-exposure. It involves avoiding a suspected food for a period of from four to twelve days and then eating a test meal of the food. Eating a masked allergen after less than four day's avoidance will simply continue the masking and the person will get no indication that the food is allergenic for him. Because of the cyclic factor some people can lose their sensitivity to a food in as little as two weeks of avoidance of it. Hence the four-to-twelve day testing period makes sure the person has avoided the food long enough to eliminate the masking, but not so long that sensitivity to it has been lost.

The reaction to the food under test conditions may not be the same as the person's usual symptoms from it. In my own case, my reaction upon testing milk was a headache, which I rarely had while drinking milk regularly. In everyday life, unmasking undoubtedly happens regularly but is not recognized as such. A person eats pistachio nuts every day or so but does not recognize that he is sensitive to them because of masking. Because of travel or illness or temporary unavailability, he isn't able to eat any for a week. Then, a little while after eating them again he finds his stomach upset. He isn't sure what caused it but feels better after awhile. Regular eating of the pistachios re-establishes the masking and he never realizes how they affect him. One can only wonder how many headaches, upset stomachs, or other temporary symptoms are the result of re-exposure to an allergenic food after accidental unmasking.

In the 1950's Randolph, based on the work of himself and Rinkel, called attention to the similarity between allergy and addiction. These doctors had observed that a patient who went without a frequently-eaten allergenic food for a period of time, ranging from a few hours to two or three days, usually felt worse from doing so, but could be relieved by eating that food again. As with addiction generally, going without the substance induces withdrawal symptoms which can be relieved by consuming more of the addictive substance. Thus we have the paradoxical fact that a person can make himself feel *better* by eating a food to which he is allergic when the allergy to that food has been masked by frequent consumption of it. This means that a person allergic to wheat, for example, is likely to note a feeling of greater well-being after having a bowl of wheat cereal or a slice of bread and never even conceive of the possibility that what makes him feel better actually is the cause of his complaints.

One woman reported on by RRZ said, "I suspect pineapple and tomato, *but I know for sure that corn and egg are agreeable because I always feel better after eating them and I eat them nearly every day.*"[5] Guess which two (and only two) foods she was sensitive to! Tomato and pineapple were innocent, causing her no symptoms.

Dr. Marshall Mandell later started linking the two terms together so that they are now used as a single concept of addictive allergy or, more commonly, allergy-addiction. As Dr. Randolph has stated: "I think of addictions and allergies as being synonyms."[6] Another clinical ecologist described it this way: "You will notice that I do not speak of allergy or addiction, but rather of a single entity— allergy/addiction. These two different aspects are as inseparable as heads and tails on a coin. Depending on which aspect is facing you, one or the other side may be more obvious but the obverse is always there."[7]

Subsequent to the publication of *Food Allergy*, Randolph also recognized that there were similarities between the body's masking response and the view of the response to stress which had been developed by Hans Selye. Starting in the 1930's Selye found, working with animals, that regardless of the nature of specific agents or conditions which put stress on the body, it responded to all stress in the same way, exhibiting a pattern Selye called the general adaptation syndrome (G.A.S.). Anything producing stress he called a stressor and used such stressors as exposure to extreme cold, injection with toxic substances and forced activity.[8]

Despite the variety of stressors, the body has only one basic response, the G.A.S., in which numerous physiological changes take place to help the body mobilize to meet the situation. One important change is an increase in activity of the adrenal glands. In the normal course of events, the need for the G.A.S. is temporary—the squirrel finding itself under attack by an eagle uses the stress produced to run as fast as it can to get away. If successful, its physiological functioning soon reverts to normal and it is then ready to meet the next threat, which may be a cold spell that the G.A.S. will help it live through.

The G.A.S. is a mobilization designed to meet an emergency. It is not intended to be a permanent way of life. During World War II, America got along for more than four years without producing any autos, radios, refrigerators, etc. for civilian use as all efforts were bent toward winning the war. We could not have continued that way indefinitely without having a breakdown in our way of life but could meet the challenge successfully for a limited period. Likewise, the body confronting a stress-producing situation responds with the G.A.S. but can not keep it up indefinitely.

Selye found that the G.A.S. followed a three-stage

pattern: (1) the alarm reaction, when the body makes the physiological changes needed to meet the threat, (2) the stage of resistance, which may be quite prolonged and when as a the result of the adaptation the body is able to handle the threat successfully, and (3) the stage of exhaustion, which occurs after the body's resources have been all used up and serious illness or death takes place.[9] During the second stage there is no outward indication of difficulty. When Selye exposed rats to extreme cold, they adjusted to it and appeared to get along normally, even showing resistance "above the normal level," but eventually they lost this ability and could not survive in even moderately cold temperatures. They had given their all.

Even when Dr. Randolph first heard of Selye's observations and theory concerning the G.A.S. in 1936 and 1937, he recognized the similarity to the response he observed in allergy patients, but it took him almost 20 years before he could make the full connection theoretically. He eventually realized why it had taken so long to do so. The physiologists who were studying laboratory animals started out with normal healthy creatures and exposed them to known stressors and followed their reactions through the three stages.

As Doctor Randolph explained it. "...we physicians didn't see patients when they were well; we hadn't known what was happening to them.... The doctors see the patients only after they get sick as they are approaching the third stage of this adaptation response, but before they get there just as their adaptation is petering off, and they begin to get sick.... Their adaptation to these common materials... begins to wane and they develop delayed recurrences of symptoms.... They are arthritic, they are asthmatic, they are psychotic, they are gastro-intestinal patients and others."[10]

Explanation of the masking response in allergy flows

readily from the G.A.S. theory. Exposure to an allergenic food regularly leads to a stage of resistance in which the body appears to be able to handle the food successfully, but sooner or later the exhaustion stage sets in and then symptoms result. Avoiding the food for at least four days eliminates the body's tolerance of it so when it is then eaten it produces an alarm reaction which can then be recognized. Also, the child who has "outgrown" its allergy is seen as one who is in the stage of resistance and when the exhaustion stage is reached the person will again have symptoms resulting from the eating the food.

The G.A.S. shows us why treatment for allergy symptoms which only covers them up with pain-killers, antihistamines, etc. not only does not correct the underlying condition but also can result in the person developing a more serious illness later on. A symptom such as an abdominal pain or a runny nose is an indication that something is not right with the body. If it results from allergy and is overpowered with drugs the person will not be led to eliminate the cause of the stress which the body is undergoing. The body will adapt as best it can but at the cost of greater stress and more severe exhaustion eventually. Then the person has real trouble.

The concepts of stress and the G.A.S. also aid in understanding why allergy can be responsible for infectious illnesses. Dr. Lendon Smith believes, for example, that "ear infections in children are basically an allergic reaction." He has concluded: "It is essentially a problem of adrenal gland exhaustion."[11] Thus allergy-caused stress leads to adrenal exhaustion which limits the ability of the body to resist infection. It is also likely that allergically irritated tissues in the ear-nose-throat area will produce more mucus and be less able to combat germs than healthy tissues. This view recognizes that germs can "cause" illness but it also takes into account that the ability of germs to do so is affected by conditions influencing the ability of the body to fight back.

In the case of allergy-addiction the body must raise its defenses anew to cope with the stress caused by each consumption of the guilty food. With an allergen consumed regularly the person has been assaulted by it so long that the emergency-level at which the body has had to keep functioning comes to seem natural to him. To go without the allergen lets the body revert to a more normal state which initially may feel uncomfortable. As with addiction generally, these feelings of discomfort can be thought of as withdrawal symptoms. Eating the allergenic food again makes the person feel better. That is why allergenic foods are likely to be one's favorites. I needed my "fix" of milk at every meal. One of my favorite foods was pancakes, which contain milk, egg, and wheat, all foods allergenic for me.

The significance of the questions at the beginning of this chapter should now be evident. The foods least likely to be allergenic for you are those in the answer to question number 5. Let us also look back to the questions mentioned in the previous chapter and see how we can now answer them.

1. *"Could it be wheat? No, I've always eaten bread and cereal and I didn't used to have these problems".* When I didn't have these problems I was in the stage of resistance and with my allergy masked there was no way of recognizing that wheat was allergenic.

2. *"How about milk? No, I tried going without that for awhile and I felt worse than ever."* I only tried going without for a couple of days and the feeling worse was the result of withdrawal symptoms.

3. *"Could it be eggs? No, I always feel better after I eat them."* A clear indication of allergy-addiction.

4. *"Could it be tuna? I felt worse after supper last night when we had tuna. No, because it didn't bother me when I*

had tuna last week." When I had tuna last week I hadn't had any before that for a month and had lost my sensitivity to it. Last week's fish set up my sensitivity to this week's fish.

Now it will be seen why the advice given me by an allergist as to how to test for milk was misleading. He said to go without it for two or three days and see how I felt. But two or three days would be the withdrawal period during which a person might well feel worse than usual. Finding that feeling worse when avoiding milk and better when drinking it would never lead one to conclude that milk was guilty without the information discussed in this chapter.

One qualification might be in order. Feeling better after eating a certain food must be interpreted in the context in which it is eaten. If you are extra hungry then almost any food could make you feel better simply because it was food, and a meal eaten in particularly satisfying social circumstances may give pleasure unrelated to the particular foods consumed. But if you feel better—more alert, happier, more energetic—after eating a certain food in an ordinary meal, then beware. Feeling the opposite way should also make one suspicious. An innocent food will not affect you very much one way or the other. A food which tastes extra good to you should also be suspect.

References

1. Rinkel, Herbert J., M.D., Randolph, Theron G., and Zeller, Michael, M.D., *Food Allergy,* Charles C. Thomas, Springfield, Ill., 1951, p. 56.

2. Hirschfeld, Herman, M.D., F.A.C.A., *The Whole Truth About Allergy,* Arco Publishing Co., 1963, pp. 134–5.

3. Rinkel, Randolph, and Zeller, op. cit., p. 116.

4. Mackarness, Richard, M.D., *Eating Dangerously,* Harcourt, Brace, Jovanovich, New York, 1976, pp. 50–51.

5. Rinkel, Randolph, and Zeller, op. cit., p. 11. emphasis in the original.

6. Challem, Jack Joseph, "An Exclusive Interview with Dr. Theron Randolph, M.D., *Bestways*, June 1977, p. 24.

7. Levin, Warren, M.D., "Allergy-Addiction to Foods and Chemicals," *Let's Live,* June 1976, p. 29.

8. Selye, Hans, M.D., *The Stress of Life,* McGraw Hill, New York, 1956, p. 30.

9. ibid., pp. 87–8.

10. Challem, op. cit., p. 24.

11. Challem, Jack Joseph, "An Exclusive Interview with 'The Children's Doctor,' Lendon H. Smith, M.D.," *Bestways,* August 1977, p. 17.

CHAPTER 5

Testing for Food Allergies

Skin Testing

WE SAW BEFORE how allergy research developed as the study of immunology. Early research found that a small amount of an allergenic substance injected just under the skin produced a local reaction with redness and swelling, the response of the body to a material to which it was sensitive. This reaction then, was diagnostic of the sensitivity; a person not sensitive to the substance, ragweed pollen for example, would show no skin reaction.

The emphasis was on airborne allergens and their manifestations in diseases such as hay fever. Following the logic of vaccination, the treatment then consisted of injecting small controlled amounts of the allergenic substance into the person at regular intervals so that the body would gradually build up a tolerance to the stuff and would become desensitized. For this kind of allergy both the methods of detection and treatment were quite successful and became standard.

Food allergy, as we have seen, is another thing. The main trouble with trying to use the immunological approach with food allergies is that it doesn't work well at all. Yet many conventional allergists still place great reliance on skin tests for food allergies. Situations are described in the medical literature in which doctors have banned many different foods from a patient's diet simply because of skin test reactions even if there was no change in symptoms after so altering the diet.

Let us take a closer look at skin tests. There are two varieties of skin test, the scratch test and the intradermal or injection type. With the scratch test a drop of solution containing the allergen to be tested is placed on the skin at the site where the skin is broken by making a scratch on it; with the intradermal test the solution is injected with a hypodermic needle just under the skin. As a control with either method, one site is given just the clear solution containing no allergen to determine the patient's reaction to the solution itself. As each test site is only a small area on the skin, a number of different substances can be tested at the same time. The degree of sensitivity to a substance is indicated by the amount of redness and swelling at the test site.

The only problem with skin tests for foods is that they are highly unreliable. Medical textbooks on allergy, whether conventional or ecological, are in considerable agreement that the accuracy of skin tests, whether scratch or intradermal, is not high. Errors may be either false positives or false negatives. That is, a skin test may indicate a sensitivity to a food where the patient shows no reaction upon eating the food or the test may show that he is not sensitive to it when in fact he is.

One conventional textbook states that "relatively few of the positive reactions are correlated with clinical sensitivity," so that positive reactions to skin tests for foods "should not be interpreted literally as indicating clinical sensitivity to the reacting foods. . . . "[1] By clinical sensitivity is meant that the patient has reactions or symptoms from eating the food, that eating it makes a difference in some way. In other words, the authors are saying that even if you have a positive skin test for a particular food, you are not likely to have any symptoms or reaction develop if you eat that food. In the unlikely event you are sensitive to a food to which you have a positive skin test reaction, you will only find out anyway by noting what happens when you actually eat the food.

Another conventional textbook similarly notes that skin tests are "useful and reasonably reliable diagnostic evidence in the study of allergy to inhaled allergens but far less reliable in the diagnosis of food allergies."[2] Feingold concurs, stating: "It is generally recognized that skin testing for foods is unreliable."[3] Crozier also minimizes the importance of skin tests for foods, maintaining that the basic means for diagnosing food allergies is the experience of the patient and noting how symptoms are affected by eating or avoiding various foods.[4]

Rinkel and his associates did a number of studies in which they compared skin test results with actual clinical sensitivity to foods as determined by feeding tests of suspect foods under unmasked conditions. One study showed that only about one fourth of positive skin tests were associated with clinical food sensitivity. In another study by Rinkel, of 659 patients, he found that the accuracy of skin tests varied somewhat according to the kind of symptom syndrome, but in no case was it higher than 40.4%.[5] For hives and gastro-intestinal conditions due to allergy, the accuracy rate was no higher than 20%. RRZ reported devastatingly that: "It is our finding that only two patients out of a hundred will give positive skin tests *to every food which* is allergenic."[6] One clinical ecologist recently ranked skin tests the least effective among a half dozen methods of ascertaining allergic food sensitivity.[7] So much for the accuracy of skin tests for food allergy.

There are a number of reasons why this should be so. For one thing, allergy can affect almost any part of the body, and the characteristics of that part may be quite different from the skin, so it is not surprising that the two respond in different ways to the substance being tested. Also, a person may be allergic to a food in its cooked state but not raw, or vice versa. Cooking alters the chemical composition of the food and may change it to something the person is or is not allergic to. A person allergic to the cooked form only would not show a reaction to a skin testing solution made from the raw form.

Another possibility is that the person might be sensitive to a product of digestion. That is, as the food is digested in the body it is altered and new chemical substances are formed. The person might be sensitive not to the food itself but to one or more of these chemical compounds formed in the digestive process. The skin test, of course, would not reveal this.

In view of all this, it is not hard to see why skin testing leaves a great deal to be desired as a means for determining food allergies. It also indicates why skin tests work relatively well for airborn allergens. These generally affect the nose and throat area whose lining is relatively similar to that of the skin. Neither would such allergens be subject to cooking or the complications of the digestive process.

Because of the great fallibility of skin tests for foods, it is easy to see why conventional allergists tend to tread lightly in this area. It would be more understandable if there were no alternatives to skin tests. It is inexcusable, however, given that research on food allergy has been published for more than 50 years and that a full-fledged highly accurate system for detecting food allergies was published more than a quarter of a century ago.

I am referring to the approach set forth in 1951 in the RRZ, *Food Allergy*. While it is now starting to receive more attention, many patients would have benefitted had this been widely adopted earlier.

The Coca Pulse Test

This is a system, mentioned earlier in this book, developed by Dr. Arthur F. Coca back in the 1930's. We noted his frustration at the failure of doctors even to investigate his system and try it and how he eventually wrote a popular book, *The Pulse Test*, which is still in print. It involves the person taking his own pulse a number of times during the day, which provided one reason for some doctors to reject the system, saying that it would make the patient too preoccupied with himself and hypochondriacal.

Many doctors charged also that Coca's method was unreliable. Sherman wrote, for example, that since the pulse is "affected by many extraneous factors, his method has gained little acceptance."[8] Although Coca does not make this clear, it is true that the pulse does not respond for all people the way he describes in his writings. I tried using his method and found that it was inconclusive for me. I was informed later by one clinical ecologist that it does not work for everyone. Yet, clinical ecologist Lawrence Dickey wrote recently: "The author has found the concept sufficiently valid to make it worthy of using in daily allergy and ecology practice."[9]

Given the limitations of skin tests, rejection of the pulse test because it is not completely reliable is indeed inconsistent. One wonders whether the failure of doctors to adopt the pulse test was really due to its unreliability or to their failure even to investigate it, which Coca repeatedly complained about. Many doctors, it seems, have a strong aversion to having the patient play a substantial role in detecting or even in understanding his own condition.

Shortly after I learned that I had an elevated blood

pressure, I had had some subjective symptoms I had experienced before and wondered if these were related to blood pressure so I stopped in our university Health Service and asked a nurse if she would check it. She informed me she couldn't do this without a doctor's approval, which so irritated me that I felt that even if I pursued the subject and got it checked the reading could be invalidated by the experience itself. Yet, blood pressure devices are widely available in mail order catalogs and even discount stores and public health officials encourage people to find out what their blood pressure is. It is said that in earlier years doctors also resisted laymen having fever thermometers and taking their own temperatures.

Given this kind of thinking it is not hard to see why there would be resistance to the pulse test. I am describing it here because it can be tried by anyone with complete safety. If it turns out not to be helpful for a person, this will become evident and all that will have been lost is the time involved. It will produce no symptoms in itself and may be used in conjunction with other approaches to be described later.

Coca got the first clue which led him to develop his method from an experience his wife had when she was given a morphine derivative for a heart condition. Instead of slowing down her pulse as expected, the rate increased greatly. Talking about the event later she mentioned that she had observed her heartbeat also increased after some meals. This led Dr. Coca to suggest that she check her pulse after eating different single foods.

Doing this revealed a number of foods which greatly accelerated her pulse over the normal amount, and she eliminated such foods from her diet. Told by two heart specialists in 1935 that she would not live more than five years, she was still alive and normally active without pain more than 20 years later. Furthermore, as she detected the allergenic foods and started avoiding them she noticed that other medical conditions cleared up.[10] Coca started using the pulse test with his allergy patients and got similarly gratifying results with them.

Anyone wishing to use this method systematically is advised to get a copy of *The Pulse Test* as I can give only some of the general guidelines here. The basic principle is that many people will have their pulse rate increased by exposure to an allergen, whether it be a food or an inhalant. Of course, other factors such as exercise or illness may increase the pulse also, so it is understood that we are talking about the pulse of a person at rest who has no illness (except allergy) that could affect the pulse.

There is a great deal of variation in pulse rates among normal people so we must view the commonly given "normal" pulse rate of 72 as being only an average. Some normal healthy people, usually joggers or athletes, may have pulse rates in the 40's and 50's. Coca found that, as people detected and avoided substances allergenic for them, their normal pulse rate usually declined somewhat. The upper limit of a normal pulse rate is more definite— 84.[11] Despite a common belief that children have fast pulses, Coca found that the pulses of normal nonallergic children were within the same range.[12]

There are two consequences of the fact that the pulse rate can be affected by airborne allergens as well as by foods. One of these is that the pulse rate can be used to test for inhalant allergens. The other is that exposure to airborne allergens after eating can make more difficult the testing of foods. This complication can be avoided by making sure that there has been no change in one's inhalant exposure after eating. The pulse generally responds quite quickly to inhalant exposure so one should avoid any new inhalant exposure for as long as one is checking the pulse to test for foods. Doing housecleaning, waxing or polishing, plumping feather pillows or making beds, going into a dusty attic or cellar, painting, etc. could all invalidate a check for food. Because tobacco is a potentially allergenic inhalant that can affect the pulse, it should be tested itself before doing other tests if one smokes or is likely to be exposed to tobacco from other people smoking while pulse testing for foods.

There is one point made by Coca that I found unsupported by other writers and misleading. He states that sensitivity to house dust "regularly excludes the commonly eaten foods as allergens."[13] This certainly was not true in my case. Other allergists emphasize the tendency to multiple sensitivities so that food and inhalant allergies are frequently found in the same person.[14]

In the absence of other explanations for a high pulse rate, allergy is a likely cause. It is not just a matter of one's pulse rate on an absolute scale but of its range during the day. Coca says the normal ranges of the resting pulse rate is 16 beats and that a greater variation than this indicates allergy even if the top figure is less than 84. A person whose pulse at some time of the day is 60, let us say, would have a normal upper limit of 76, anything above that indicating allergy.

It is not hard to take one's own pulse. The most common site is at the wrist just up the arm about an inch and a half from the base of the thumb. A little hollow spot will be found with the finger tips. One should not press too hard. The pulse may also be felt on the side of the head just in front of the ear about even with the ear opening. Accuracy is important and Coca stresses counting for a full minute using the second hand of a watch or clock and not just counting, say, for 15 seconds and then multiplying by four.

A substantial rise in the rate after getting up in the morning but before eating breakfast may be due to an allergen in toothpaste or some cosmetic item. The pulse rate is not affected by masking so there is no need to avoid the substance for several days before testing.

Anyone using this method, as well as any other system that involves noting reactions to exposures to possible allergens, is strongly advised to keep a detailed diary. In this case it would include every food that was eaten and the pulse rates before and after as will be described shortly. It would also be a good idea to note possible other causes of a pulse rate variation such as exposure to paint fumes, dusty old papers, etc. In more complicated cases, reviewing the diary periodically could help one to spot likely sources of an allergic reaction.

Generally, one's pulse rate will be at its lowest just after awakening in the morning. If it is lower at any other period in the day, this points to house dust allergy, bedding being a particularly good source of house dust. Regardless of the time of the day at which the lowest pulse rate is observed, the nonallergic range should not exceed 16 beats above that.

Coca suggests two ways in which the pulse test may be employed. One is in the testing of single foods. The pulse is counted in the morning before arising and then again just before eating the first food tested. The pulse is taken 30 minutes after eating the food and again at 60 minutes. Then another food may be eaten followed by 30-minute and 60-minute pulse countings, and so on. [15] Although he does not say so I would think it better to delay trying another food if the 60-minute pulse is still elevated from the preceding food. Any abnormal increase in the pulse rate is indicative of allergy.

The other method involves keeping track of the pulse both before and after full normal meals. If one's pulse is 70 just before eating and it does not go above 84 in the next hour and a half one may conclude that that meal did not include any allergenic foods. Coca recommends taking the pulse just before and 30, 60, and 90 minutes after eating.[16] If the pulse does go up abnormally after the meal then this means either the foods in that meal should be tested individually or that other meals including some of the same foods may be looked at to see what foods are common to every pulse-raising meal.

Keep in mind the principles of food sensitivity mentioned in the preceding chapter as these apply to the pulse test also. If a cyclic allergenic food has not been eaten for awhile, the person may have lost sensitivity to it, so to be sure of the test results one should have eaten that food within the preceding two weeks. Also, not just major foods but incidental ones such as gravies, sauces and spices may be allergenic and may complicate the interpretation not just of this method but of any involving noting reactions to eating.

I mentioned that the pulse test was inconclusive for me. While my pulse went into the 90's and over 100 at times there did not seem to be any consistency to it. A food which seemed to be responsible for a rise at one time did not give the same reaction another day. Foods which I found out later I was definitely allergic to did not result in an unusual increase in pulse rate. (I still have the daily records I kept while trying the pulse test.) I am including a discussion of the method here despite my personal experience with it because it apparently has been effective for many people.

Elimination and Escalation Diets

These are two methods developed by allergists back in the 1930's and are still the basic means used by most doctors today to track down food sensitivities. It was these that I had in mind when I wrote about my own allergy experience in Chapter 2, and said that by 1940 the means to detect the cause of my difficulties had been developed and published. Both methods involve having the person eat only a limited number of foods and noting the consequences.

The escalation diet, which is the older of the two, starts out with only one food and has the patient add a new food every four to seven days and watch for symptoms that may develop as each new food is added.[17] One drawback to this method will immediately suggest itself—the difficulty and monotony of sustaining such a limited diet over the months it would take to test enough foods to get back to something approaching a more normal eating pattern.

With what we now know about the variations that people exhibit in their tolerance to foods, another problem becomes evident. People with low inherant tolerance could actually become sensitized to a previously tolerated food simply from eating it as frequently as would be required in the early stages of the testing. With only one or a few foods permitted toward the beginning of the diet, the person would wind up eating the same food again and again. RRZ reported a case where a woman became allergic within one week to foods she had previously tolerated, simply because she ate these "safe" foods repeatedly during that time.[18] Newly acquired sensitivity would also interfere with the interpretation of the test. Symptoms would most frequently develop only after several days of exposure, by which time another food would have been added, which would then probably be blamed for the symptoms. The escalator diet, then, is not the ultimate answer to food allergy detection.

The elimination diet, associated with the name of Dr. Albert Rowe, takes a different approach. The patient is given a list of only a relatively small number of foods and is told to eat only those on the list, and, of course, to note what results these foods may produce. After two or three weeks the patient consults with the doctor and is given another list containing a different group of foods to eat.

The process is repeated until all the relevant foods have been tested. This process is somewhat more workable than the escalation diet and can be used with a fair degree of success by a determined doctor and patient.

The elimination diet is the method most commonly used by conventional allergists, although with a considerable amount of individual variation. As one recent author described it, "Every allergist conducts an elimination diet somewhat different from the way others do it. All that is required is that the food be eliminated completely and for a long enough time to see if such removal is accompanied by relief of . . . symptoms."[19] He adds that confirmation comes from seeing if symptoms reappear when the food is reinstated.

What this amounts to is that the food group approach of the elimination diet gives either an OK or a warning for a number of foods at one time. If the person has no trouble from eating foods in Group A, but does with Group B, then he or she can eat the foods in Group A while those in Group B are added to the diet one at a time as in the escalator system to isolate the guilty one or ones. Meanwhile, the patient has the variety in his diet permitted by knowing a number of foods that can be tolerated by him.

There are still limitations with this approach though. If each group of foods tested, or even a few such groups each happen to contain even one food which is allergenic for the person, then detection will be very difficult. For the majority of people who may have only a few sensitivities the method may work fine. The low tolerance person susceptible to many allergens could find the elimination method a long, drawn out, inconvenient process that might not ultimately be successful. While not as severe as with the escalator diet, there could still be the problem of new sensitivities developing from repeated consumption of a limited number of foods.

Also, some allergens could be missed in the procedure, as in the following situation. A person has a cyclic sensitivity to potato, which is dropped from his diet as he tries out other foods, and he improves. Because of the testing process it is two or three months before he gets back to potato. By that time he has lost his sensitivity to it, notices no initial symptoms and so resumes eating it. Masking develops so he gets no immediate reaction from eating it but his symptoms eventually return. He knows that he improved after dropping the group containing potato, yet every food in the group appeared to be innocent after being re-introduced singly. Eventually he or his doctor may stumble on the answer but only after great difficulty. He may just as likely conclude that his trouble must not be allergy and either gives up hope of finding the cause of his trouble or begins a round of seeing other medical specialists.

RAST

There are some recently developed other possible ways of testing for allergy that may be used by clinical ecologists. One of these is RAST—Radio Allergo-Sorbent Test. This involves testing for antibodies to different foods by means of analysis of a sample of blood from the patient. Advantages are that more than one substance may be tested using the same blood sample and that the test takes place in a laboratory and does not involve producing a reaction within the patient's body. Disadvantages are that it is relatively expensive and that, because it is concerned only with immunological antibodies, it does not detect all allergens. The interpretation of test results is clear-cut, however, unlike that of skin tests. A positive result, i.e., finding antibodies to a certain food, definitely indicates sensitivity to that food. A negative result is not decisive but can be confirmed by checking the food in an eating test.

Provocative Testing

The most effective tests are those that most closely duplicate the exposures the person actually encounters in everyday life. Because these tests deliberately seek to provoke a response in the person to a suspected allergen, they are referred to as provocative tests. A number of clinical ecologists use sublingual or intradermal provocative tests, in which a food or chemical extract of known strength is either injected into the patient or dropped just under the tongue. If the person is sensitive to the substance he will usually have a reaction similar to one which would result from actually consuming it. The procedure is quite different from the conventional skin tests which, assuming that they work, only produce a generalized reaction on the skin at the site of the test. If there is a reaction to the extract in a provocative test, it will ordinarily take place within a few minutes and can usually be terminated by use of a dilute solution of that extract, so that quite a number of foods and chemicals can be tested in a single day. Even these tests are not infallible, the ultimate test being the eating of a food and noting whether there is a reaction to it.

The major problem in getting clinical ecology testing is the limited number of clinical ecologists. One can get help in locating one by writing: The Society for Clinical Ecology, c/o Del Stigler, M.D., 2205 Franklin, Suite 490, Denver, Colorado 08215. According to information given me by Dr. Marshall Mandell, an official of the society, there are about 200 members, but not all of them are fully active in clinical ecology. Even of those who are, some have their practices limited to medical specialties such as pediatrics or psychiatry that would be inappropriate for many people. Thus, in the whole United States there are only a relatively small number of clinical ecologists available. The number is increasing, however, as more doctors find out about the field and begin to use a clinical ecology approach in their work. But if all those who read this book were to seek out clinical ecologists, they would be overwhelmed.

Those who do not have ready access to a clinical ecologist may wish to consider testing on a do-it-yourself basis, perhaps in cooperation with one's family doctor. For the majority of people this would no doubt be a realistic workable alternative. Persons with certain conditions that will be mentioned shortly, however, should observe the cautions specified. In any event, one should not do any testing until after having read this whole book. A number of points will be mentioned later on that one should know before testing. Diabetics, for example, will want to be familiar with the material in Chapter 8.

The testing methods to be described involve the deliberate production of an allergic reaction, and while this is generally no more than what the person might experience as a result of particular circumstances in everyday life, occasionally the responses can be severe to the point of needing medical attention. There are certain types of people who definitely should *not* undertake provocative testing without assurance of being able to get immediate medical assistance. These are:[20]

1). Asthmatics.

2). Epileptics.

3). Diabetics on insulin.

4). Those in a "markedly debilitated state".

5). People suffering from or subject to severe emotional disturbance.

6). Anyone who has had an allergic reaction strong enough to have required medical attention in the past.

These same qualifications apply to the fasting test to be described shortly. With individuals who are very susceptible, both the withdrawal of food during a fast and its reintroduction during testing can precipitate an asthmatic or epileptic attack, or for those with psychotic or severe neurotic tendencies, a period of irrationality and lack of insight. Such psychological reactions following the eating of a food after a period of avoidance will usually be brief—an hour or so—but in rare cases can last up to three days. The temporary distress will be balanced by the knowledge that a food causing serious trouble for the person has been discovered. One should not panic and have the person put in a mental hospital where he or she might be given a diet containing allergenic foods which would maintain the condition.

While these cautions should make one aware of possible hazards for the kinds of individuals specified, they are certainly not intended to discourage others from using provocative testing. Randolph has had experience with over 50,000 individual feeding tests during his career, a good part of them at home, and other doctors have used them also, Dr. Lawrence Dickey in Colorado having used home tests for some 30 years.[21] While Randolph gave some of his patients medical assistance because of their reactions to the test, he has reported that he never has had a death or irreversible complication result from testing.[22]

This information on provocative testing is not given with the expectation that everyone will try it on a do-it-yourself basis. Rather, it is recommended that the reader seek out a doctor and do the testing under medical supervision. It need not necessarily be an allergist, for the concern is with an acute allergic reaction, which any doctor should be able to handle, so if there is no allergist conveniently available and your family doctor agrees to cooperate, that should be quite adequate.

For reasons which we have looked at earlier, your doctor, whether allergist or otherwise, may not be familiar with provocative testing. While I will describe the procedure here, he may wish to do more reading in the medical literature. The best source for the single-food eating test would still be the Rinkel-Randolph-Zeller book, *Food Allergy*. This book has been out of print for a number of years, but Dr. Marshall Mandell has arranged to have it reprinted through the New England Foundation for Allergic and Environmental Diseases, 3 Brush Street, Norwalk, Connecticut 06850. Copies may be ordered by writing to the foundation at that address. A brief description of testing procedures is contained in *Ecologic Medicine Manual* by William H. Philpott, M.D., a mimeographed booklet which may be ordered from his clinic, Ecology House and Clinic and Laboratory, 820 N.E. 63rd Street, Oklahoma City, Oklahoma, 73105. A thorough treatment of the whole field of clinical ecology including provocative food testing is in a medical textbook, *Clinical Ecology*, by Lawrence D. Dickey, M.D. (Charles C. Thomas, publisher, Springfield, Illinois). Information on testing may also be found in *A Physician's Handbook on Orthomolecular Medicine*, by Roger J. Williams, M.D. and Dwight K. Kalita, Ph.D. (Pergamon Press, New York.).

A number of doctors unfortunately are quite authoritarian and would refuse to get involved with an unfamiliar procedure. Some doctors resent it when a patient appears to know more about a subject than they do. If you cannot get the cooperation of a doctor, should you try provocative testing on your own? Only you can answer that question for yourself. If you have had medical problems which you have not been able to get resolved with conventional medical treatment, you may have little hesitation in deciding to go ahead. There was no doubt in my mind but that I wanted to do the testing. But if any one of the six cautions mentioned on page 88 applies to you, then you certainly should not do food tests without being sure that you could get medical attention quickly if needed for an allergic reaction.

The great majority of people, however, will have no trouble and consider that temporary symptoms are a price they would gladly pay to find out the cause of their suffering. As Mackarness stated: "The most striking thing about this unmasking of food allergies is the satisfaction with which patients suddenly recognize their old, familiar symptoms for what they are: simple reactions to the food they have been eating. . . . It is heartening to know the cause of an illness and be able to do something about it, instead of wondering whether you are a freak. . . ."[23]

The Food-Activities-and-Symptoms Diary

Whether done in cooperation with a doctor or not, it is strongly recommended that a food-activities-and-symptom diary be kept. If you fast or have a test week of unusual foods, as will shortly be described, it would be a good idea to begin the diary a week or two beforehand. The diary should note each food that you have, some indication as to amount, and the time of the day. Any prepared food should include the brand name; you may wish to check back later on the ingredients as listed on the label. Remember to record incidental foods like olives or pickles, salad dressings and seasonings. Be sure to include all snacks during the day and evening. Anything you drink besides water should also be recorded.

Your diary should also include the activities you engage in. This could help to locate nonfood allergens which could be giving you trouble. Unless you do exactly the same thing at exactly the same place every day at work, record your different tasks and where you did them at work. You might find out, for example, that you notice certain symptoms after you have used the office copier or have been to a certain part of the plant or handled a certain type of material. Likewise, write down the different jobs you do around home—cutting the grass, waxing the floors or working down in the basement.

Lastly, the diary should note any symptoms that you have such as a runny nose, nausea, irritability, pains, etc. and when you have them. Kept over a period of time a diary can be very helpful in isolating the cause of reactions in difficult cases. If you have a certain symptom, say headaches, reviewing a diary that has been kept over a period of time should show what exposure has usually preceded the headache. Although inhalants usually produce their effects quickly, keep in mind that foods sometimes can have delayed reactions, so that the symptom you experience one day may be the result of something eaten the day before. Check the foods eaten the day before the symptom was noticed if there seems to be nothing you can discover on the same day.

There is another possible reason for variations in symptoms that should be mentioned. A person exposed to an allergen every day or so may develop a pattern, as I did, of a regular cycle of getting better and worse. In my case the cycle repeated itself about every three weeks. I have concluded that this was an alternation between the adaption and exhaustion stages of the G.A.S. I would have a strong onset of symptoms which gradually receded until I was almost up to normal, only to have the whole process repeat itself. While an extra-large amount of my most powerful allergen, milk, might start the cycle anew, I believe now that even though the symptoms varied over a period of time this was due more to changes in the ability of my body to adapt to a constantly-recurring allergen than to differential exposure to the allergen itself. After dropping milk from my diet, I have found it much easier to note the specific effects of other foods. But a food-activities-and-symptoms diary should help you to spot such a cyclic pattern also.

Fasting and the Uncommon Foods Test

There are two ways of testing, either of which will show within a few days whether any problems you might be having are being caused by food allergy. If the results are negative, then you will need to start considering other alternatives, although inhalant or contact allergies would still be possibilities. If you are having regular trouble as a result of food allergy, it should be evident from what we have seen that this must be due to one or more foods which are eaten frequently, i.e., at least every two or three days. Hence, to see if allergy is a cause, one avoids all of these frequently-eaten foods for from four to six days to see if this makes a difference. Skin disturbances might not clear up within this time but most other conditions due to allergy should definitely improve.

The most clear-cut test is to go without any food during this time, but drinking water as desired. The idea of fasting has gotten much more widely accepted in recent years than it was in the past, so that a proposal to go without food for a few days will not seem very unusual to many readers. Fasting is not that hard for the average person. After the second day of the fast, sensations of hunger usually become minimal and most people feel as though they are "coasting." The pulse rate is likely to decrease. Some fasters find that they feel light-headed for a moment if they rise quickly from a seated or lying position; all that is needed in such cases is either to stand up more slowly or to pause briefly after arising until normal circulation is re-established and the feeling passes. Because tap water may contain allergens, as noted in an earlier chapter, it would be best if either distilled or spring water would be used during the fast.

It will help in clearing trouble-causing food residues from the system to take two tablespoonsfull of unflavored milk of magnesia just at the beginning of the fast.[24] If you have food allergy, the test fast will surely reveal it. Ordinarily by the fourth day a person will definitely feel better and allergy-caused symptoms—headaches, gastrointestinal, muscular, nasal, emotional, or whatever—should be markedly reduced or eliminated. Mandell reported on a woman who had many severe symptoms and needed 10 days for all of them to clear, but by the fifth day some of them had started to ease so that she could note improvement. This was a definite indication to continue the fast. She had been instructed by Dr. Mandell to drink two quarts of spring water each day and was permitted to take natural sea salt as desired. Some people have a feeling of greater energy while fasting than while eating.

Because of the addiction-withdrawal phenomenon, however, one might feel worse or even somewhat ill on the second or third day. This in itself would be evidence of food allergy-addiction. On the third day of the fast of the woman mentioned above, not only did her old symptoms continue but also new ones developed—pain at the site of a 20-year old operation, upper back pain and cramps in both legs. Withdrawal symptoms may be eased by taking a heaping teaspoon of a mixture of two parts sodium bicarbonate and one part potassium bicarbonate in an eight-ounce glass of water followed by a second glass of water for up to four times per day.[25]

If you do not feel better by the fourth day, try continuing the fast for two or three more days. If you notice no changes after a week it is highly unlikely that whatever is causing your trouble is food allergy. The woman we have been describing reported to Dr. Mandell: "On the tenth morning I was free of all my former symptoms but very tired and weak. All of my doubts concerning fasting and the underlying nature of my many ailments finally were gone and, for the first time in many years, I was able to stop worrying about the prolonged downward course of my health. My response to fasting was like a miracle! An important part of my diagnosis was now very clear because we had completely eliminated every complaint that I had suffered from for the past 10 years. All of that misery had been unnecessary and could have been avoided because it was due to controllable exposures to environmental substances that I reacted to."[26]

It should be noted that this woman took precautions to minimize her exposure to potential nonfood allergens during her fast. Aerosol sprays, perfumed cosmetics, disinfectants, laundry bleaches, household waxes and polishes, etc. were removed from the home during the fast (see the chapter on chemical allergens) and no smoking, painting or use of nail polish or removers was permitted.[27]

If you do not wish to undergo a fast, then there is another alternative which, while not as sure as a fast, will probably work for most people. Start by making a list of every food and beverage you consume at least once every three days whether at regular meals or between-meals and bedtime snacks. Include coffee, tea, alcoholic or soft drinks if these are ordinarily taken. If you regularly eat certain processed foods such as breakfast cereals, egg substitutes, meat extenders, etc. read their labels to find all the foods included in them and put the basic food type ("corn meal," for example) on your list. You will have to disregard the ingredients with chemical names unless you happen to be a dietician or food chemist. Monosodium glutamate (MSG) may be made from either wheat, corn or beets. Ham, bacon, and most lunch meats will have some corn from their processing.

You may be surprised at how short your list is, but whatever its length it contains all the foods you should *not* eat for at least a week. The idea is for one week to eat foods you do not ordinarily eat thus avoiding exposure to your most likely food allergens. During the test week do not eat any factory-prepared foods that come in cans or boxes. Also do not eat in restaurants. Even as simple a food as a restaurant steak could have seasonings which could throw you off.

Confine yourself to foods mainly from the produce section but with simple frozen foods also permitted. If you eat a food on one day do not have it again for three days. This may mean that you largely repeat your first day menu on the fourth day, etc. The idea is to avoid repeated exposure to any one food and to limit the foods to those not ordinarily eaten. Avoid seasonings even if the food tastes flat, although table salt is all right. A little sugar could be used. It should be of a type different from what you normally use; if you usually use cane sugar then try beet sugar, or vice versa. Vary your sweetening with honey, or pure maple syrup (not just maple-flavored syrup) or a sugar substitute. As with fasting it would be a good idea to use bottled water rather than tap water for drinking (and for cooking if the water is absorbed by or is served with the food).

You can include foods you eat ordinarily but not frequently. Thus, if you eat carrots only about once a week and sweet potatoes once a month you could include them in your test week diet. Try as much as possible, though, to eat foods you ordinarily never have. Look over parts of the produce counter you usually pass by. Try some uncommon meats or seafoods. This may increase your costs but after all it is only for a week. Ready-made salad dressings would be out, of course, because of their numerous ingredients but you could experiment with some simple dressings. Olive oil and lemon juice together can made a satisfactory dressing for one day.

Because of possible cross-sensitivities it would be best to avoid all the cereal grains during the week. If you feel you need the food value of cereal, restrict yourself to those not ordinarily eaten. This might include rice or oats. More likely would be millet or buckwheat. The latter two are available in health food stores. Both take a half hour to cook as a cereal; use one part of millet to three of water, with buckwheat one part to two parts of water.

The many different kinds of nuts offer other possibilities. So that you can keep from eating the same kind every day without having to buy large amounts of each of them, you could get mixed nuts and pick out different kinds on different days. Peanuts are members of the legume family which includes peas, lentils and beans. Also, do not overlook seeds such as those of sesame, pumpkin and sunflower.

If there are foods you know or suspect you are sensitive to, you should of course see that they are avoided during the uncommon foods test. The goal is to try to avoid as much as possible any foods to which you are likely to react. You may or may not like the things you try or are limited to for the week, but taste is not the object. The alternative would be to eat nothing. You may not get a balanced diet. You certainly won't if you fast! But nutritional needs can be set aside for a few days in the interest of tracking down guilty foods. You may stumble across a food to which you have a permanent sensitivity and get some kind of reaction from it. If it was eaten with several other foods at a meal, you may not be able to identify the offender at the time, but after the uncommon foods test period you could check individually each of the foods eaten at that meal to determine the troublemaker. The fact of having gotten a reaction to a food would in itself be significant in pointing to your susceptibility to food allergy.

If you go about this test right, you should be successful in avoiding all your regular food allergens. As with a fast, if food allergy is your problem you should feel better by the end of the week. If you do not, your alternatives are either to try a complete fast or to conclude that you are not allergic to foods. If you have really avoided all your usual foods the latter conclusion would be the more likely. At the end of either the fast or the uncommon foods test you are already prepared for testing foods.

Testing Procedures

Both methods of provocative testing which will be described require that there has been no ingestion of the food to be tested for at least four days, but that it should have been consumed within 12 days of the test. At least four days avoidance are required so that the body will let down the defenses which maintain the masking process. After 12 days some people can have lost their sensitivity to the food.

It is possible to meet the needs of these testing procedures without either fasting or making the uncommon foods test. They were described as a way of quickly determining whether food allergy is a factor in your case. If you are sure it is or do not want to make such a general test, you may simply start in testing individual foods, but of course you must still observe the four-to-12 day limitations mentioned just above.

In any event remember that avoiding the food for four days means *complete* avoidance, which means eating no foods that you do not know the complete contents of which means no factory or restaurant-prepared foods. At the

beginning of the process *everything* is suspect. This includes any vitamins or medications. If you are taking prescribed medicine, you should check with your doctor to see if he would agree to your stopping it for a few days. If he does not consent, then you should try to find out all the ingredients in the medication. You need to be concerned not just with the active ingredients in medicines but also with possible inert substances—flavorings, the liquid containing the medication, binders or fillers used to hold tablets together, etc. Similarly, one may be sensitive either to vitamins or to inert ingredients in the tablets, so these should be avoided for a period and then tested like foods.*
Toothpaste may also contain allergens; the presence of corn as an ingredient in some toothpastes has already been mentioned. Flavorings or other ingredients may also affect some people. Toothpaste can be avoided by using a mixture of salt and baking soda for brushing. Then note if any reactions follow resumption of use of your toothpaste.

With the cereal grains and legumes, it would probably be best to avoid all members of each family for the four days prior to testing one of their members. Thus, eating rye or barley could keep alive the masking for wheat which would appear upon testing to be innocent. Peas, beans and peanuts could work similarly.

All of these cautions may make you feel overwhelmed. That is good. It shows that you have a proper respect for the trouble-causing possibilities of the foods in your environment. In my own case I remember the feelings of discomfort when I got to the point, just as I was ready to begin testing, where everything was suspect and each food I looked at had to be thought of as, "Maybe you're the troublemaker." It can shake a person's feelings of

---

*Chelated minerals and time-release vitamin preparations are likely to contain a greater number of ingredients and hence offer a greater chance of containing an ingredient to which a person could be sensitive.

confidence, but so can a constant series of illnesses.

There is an additional consideration for someone who smokes. Aside from its other characteristics, tobacco can be an allergen for some people, and for these tobacco could complicate the interpretation of fasting and testing results. For this reason a smoker should abstain during a fast or during the period of avoiding common foods. After four days of absence from tobacco, it can then be tested as an allergen. There are two methods that can be used, either of which may produce an unpleasant reaction for the susceptible individual. Philpott recommends testing by "chain smoking as fast as possible a maximum of six cigarettes," after the four days of avoidance.[28] Feelings of nausea or dizzyness resulting from this test indicate an allergy to tobacco as not all people will be affected in this fashion. The other method is a sublingual test which will be described shortly. There actually is another way which might reveal allergy to tobacco, using the pulse test to check the pulse before and after smoking, an appreciable rise in the pulse rate pointing to allergy. However, I am assuming that anyone using either of the two methods to be described next has found the pulse test not to be completely satisfactory and so would need one of these two.

Sublingual Testing

This is a faster method than the individual deliberate feeding test to be described shortly. The drawback is that sublingual testing is not as accurate, but unlike skin tests, the inaccuracy is not random and you will know clearly where you stand. Any positive reaction (any type of symptom or response) to a sublingual test is definite evidence of sensitivity to that substance, and means that it should be avoided—at least for a few months when it can be checked again to see if sensitivity to it has been lost. If it has, the food can be re-introduced into the diet cautiously as discussed in an earlier chapter. One may have no reaction to a sublingual test and yet be sensitive to the food, so that while a positive reaction always indicates sensitivity, a negative reaction is not conclusive.

The sublingual provocative food test is based on the fact that blood vessels under the tongue are very thin and close to the surface so that anything there will be absorbed directly and quickly into the bloodstream. This principle is used for administering some types of medicines, as with nitroglycerine pills for heart patients. As used in clinical ecology, a small amount of an extract of a food or chemical is placed under the tongue and the reactions are noted. They will generally be the same as if the substance itself had been consumed. Reactions generally show up within a half hour and subside fairly quickly. Stronger or longer lasting reactions can frequently be turned off by administering a dilute solution of the same extract.

As done in the offices of clinical ecologists, sublingual testing is a precise procedure. The exact composition of the extracts are known and their potencies are carefully determined. Different strengths of the extract can be used successively in the testing procedure, and the dilution of the turnoff dose can be accurately established. Except for the development of an occasional strong reaction necessitating a temporary cessation of testing, a new substance can be tested every 30 to 45 minutes. Chemicals can be tested as well as foods.

There is no way the person at home can hope to approach the precision and variety of clinical ecologists' sublingual testing methods. However, in circumstances where the person simply cannot arrange to see a clinical ecologist, a crude form of sublingual testing can be done at home. One would need the help of a friend or relative; this is not really the sort of thing a person can do alone.

You start with small amounts of each food to be tested, each food being in a clean cup or glass. (Plastic or paper containers should be avoided as some people could be sensitive to substances in them the food would absorb.) As described by Mackarness, the food is prepared as follows: "Each sample is dropped into an electric blender, which must be absolutely free of all other food residues. Just enough distilled water to cover the rotating blades is added, and food and water are blended into a concentrated solution thin enough to be drawn up into a dropper syringe."[29] Several foods can be prepared, each placed in a clean cup or glass and labeled. If a food is eaten in both cooked and raw forms a separate solution may be prepared for each form.

Before the test the person administering it should make careful observation of the testee, taking into account psychological state, color of skin, pulse rate, the eyes (noting the size of the pupils), degree of restlessness, etc. Subjective reports of the testee will also help—any feelings regarding the stomach, whether the nose is stuffy or runny, sensations in the mouth or throat, headache, feelings of alertness, any sensations regarding other parts of the body, etc. The testee should be in a fairly normal condition to start with or reactions produced by the test may not be distinguished from the other symptoms.

The testee tilts his head back holding his mouth open with the tongue touching the roof of the mouth. The tester, using a syringe or medicine dropper, quickly places one or two drops under the testee's tongue. "The patient keeps his mouth open for two minutes, then brings his head forward and rinses his mouth with distilled water."[30] The pulse is then taken, a definite increase in rate or a considerable change in the strength of the pulse indicating an allergic sensitivity to the food, although some people can get reactions without it affecting the pulse.

Regardless of pulse the tester should look for any change which takes place in the testee, comparing with the observations made before the test—changes in skin color, size of eye pupil either increasing or decreasing, behavior of the person, etc. As soon as it is clear that the person has gotten a reaction from the food, the "turnoff" process may be started.

The idea of turnoff is to use a dilute solution of the food being tested to bring an end to the reaction. The simplest way is to use a 10 milliliter (ml.) marked syringe. With one ml. of the original testing solution in the syringe, enough distilled water is drawn into it to make a total of 10 ml. The test solution has thus been diluted to one-tenth its original strength. Shake the syringe to make sure the dilution is evenly mixed and then put one or two drops of this diluted solution under the testee's tongue. If this does not end the reaction, then repeat the process by squirting all but one ml. of the dilution out of the syringe and then drawing in enough water to again make a total of 10 ml. but this time squirting all but one ml. under the testee's tongue. In infrequent cases the dilution and squirting procedure may need to be repeated one or two more times.

If an unmarked syringe or medicine dropper is used, it would probably be better to mix up the dilutions ahead of time using other containers such as cups or small glasses. Ten ml. equals approximately two teaspoonsful. Depending on just what you used to measure with, it might be easier to get more accurate proportions if you mixed up larger quantities than you would actually use, one teaspoon of the testing solution to three tablespoons of water, for example, for the first dilution. Some of this could then be used for making the second dilution, and so on. Even if the dilutions would not be needed it would be better to have them available rather than trying to mix them up in the middle of the testing procedure.

In addition to the fact that a home-prepared testing solution would not be of a known strength, there is the possibility, mentioned to me by Dr. Mandell, that the substance in the food which causes trouble for a particular person might not be dissolved out into the solution during the brief time interval between the solution's preparation and administration. Commercial extracts, he pointed out, may be many days in preparation, with glycerine also being used to dissolve out all possible soluble substances. Thus, a home-prepared mixture would be comparatively quite crude and incomplete. The main effect of this, though, would be to produce a higher proportion of false negative results compared to commercial extracts. But sublingual testing is primarily a screening procedure with the final answer for negative results being the eating of the food in question. Mackarness used home-prepared solutions with quite satisfactory results with his patients in England.

While reactions to sublingual testing generally show up fairly soon, it is possible to get a delayed reaction. It may not be possible to turn off every reaction that does develop even using commercial extracts. The first day I visited Dr. Mandell's clinic, a woman had a reaction to a safflower oil test that affected her for a good part of the day. Despite her temporary discomfort produced by the test, she was certainly far ahead to have discovered a food which would affect her so strongly.

Dr. H.L. Newbold, a New York City clinical ecologist, has made a movie showing sublingual tests being given to some of his patients in a group testing situation. For some reason, all the patients shown were attractive young women, leading doctors in Rome, where he showed the film, to ask if that was the only kind of patient he had.

As mentioned earlier, tobacco may be an allergen for some people and if the pulse test does not work for a person, tobacco may be tested sublingually. As described by Mackarness, the smoker should abstain from smoking for five days and then prepare a testing solution by having a friend blow smoke (perhaps using a drinking straw) through a small amount of water until the solution is brown. The response may be strong: "One drop of this solution under the tongue will often bring a reaction so devastating that the addict will never wish to smoke again."[31]

The Individual Deliberate
Food Test

There is no surer way of finding out whether a particular food is allergenic for a person than by individual food testing under unmasked conditions. The first use of this method of testing was by Rinkel in 1933,[32] and the system was well developed when reported on by RRZ in *Food Allergy* in 1951. At that time they did their testing in the middle of the day, having their patients come into the office and eat the food being tested where they could be observed both before the meal and for two hours afterward. After the initial testing was done and the patient understood the principles of food testing, additional testing could be done at home.

Now, sublingual testing makes it possible for clinical ecologists to screen for trouble-causing foods much more rapidly, but as we have seen, verification by eating the food is still necessary. The majority of patients at present can be treated satisfactorily with a combination of sublingual testing (with the particular substances that are tested depending upon an evaluation of the person's background and likely sensitivities) followed by a recommended diet program. The latter will, initially at least, have an element of testing to it as the person eats questionable foods under unmasked conditions.

Where the circumstances warrant medically supervised individual deliberate feeding tests, present procedures are somewhat different from earlier ones. Whereas earlier patients were asked simply to abstain from the food to be tested for four days beforehand, the present approach is to have them fast before testing, a practice initiated by Dr. Randolph at the suggestion of Dr. Donald Mitchell of Canada. Dr. Randolph also has such patients hospitalized where other possible troublemakers such as chemical pollutants can be minimized (see the section on comprehensive environmental control in a later chapter). There also has been a tendency to increase the number of foods tested per day; Dr. Harris Hosen of Port Arthur, Texas does up to six food tests in a day.[33] Doing more tests per day reduces the time, cost and inconvenience to the patient.

Dr. Mandell made the case to me that from the standpoint of health and long-range well being it is well worth it to a person to take the time and money necessary to consult a clinical ecologist and learn of one's sensitivities and how to deal with them. Certainly, that is the best approach. If there is not such a doctor in one's community though, and if one has commitments which preclude a stay out of town, or for various other reasons one wants to try testing on one's own, information about doing so will be given here.

There is the question of when to do the testing. It would not be a good idea to eat a test food just before or during work. A reaction to the food would be inconvenient at work, and demands of the job could keep one from being able to observe adequately the effects of the test food. An evening meal would be a possibility—Mackarness uses this—but one would need to keep awake and observant for several hours afterward. One alternative would be to try testing only on weekends or other days off when three or four foods could be tested during the day. For the same reasons as with working, one should not try to combine testing with a vigorous schedule of activities around home. Also, one should avoid doing things that would involve contacts with potential nonfood allergens such as paint, wax, dusty bedding, glues, perfumes and cosmetics, etc.

Observe closely how you feel before eating the food as you will want to notice whether any changes occur afterward. You should be relatively quiet both before and after eating so that there is a full opportunity to note the effects of the food. For the test meal nothing but the food being tested should be eaten except that a little sea salt can be used if desired. The object is testing, not tasting. For the test, a normal portion of the food is eaten. If there is no reaction within an hour, then a half-portion of it is then eaten.[34]

The particular foods you test will depend upon what you think are likely troublemakers for you. Certainly you should test all foods ordinarily eaten at least once every three days. These would probably include the foods most commonly found to be allergenic as described earlier. Philpott starts with the cereal grains, taking wheat first. If there is no reaction to wheat he tests it again. "Wheat continues to be tested until there is evidence of a reaction even if it takes four meals a day for three days."[35] Only after getting no reaction from all this will he conclude that wheat is safe for that person. Most doctors are not this extreme, and it is not surprising that he finds a higher proportion of his patients to be wheat-sensitive than do other doctors.

Philpott has found that some of the most severe reactions to wheat occur on the second or third day of testing it. If you do not test wheat this thoroughly at first and get no reaction from it, but are still having trouble after ruling out other foods, you may wish to retest wheat more extensively. Of course, wheat may produce a reaction as a result of the first test meal. After testing wheat, Philpott goes on to test mature corn (corn meal), fresh corn, oats and rice in that order. He does not test rye and barley because of their similarity to wheat, concluding that a person will respond in the same way to all three.

The repetitive feeding used by Philpott for wheat is based on the finding, reported on by RRZ, that in some cases a food will not produce a reaction after just a single eating, but that it may have to be consumed several times in a row to produce an effect. RRZ termed this a cumulative reaction.[36] It is relatively uncommon, however. It might be that in such cases immediate reactions are so subtle that they are not noticed.

In my case I got no particular reactions after eating wheat under test conditions for two meals, but the next morning I woke up with a feeling like a mild sore throat which went away during the day. Wheat is tested as a cooked cereal (Ralston's, Wheatena or Cream of Wheat) or cold (puffed wheat or shredded wheat). Other wheat cereals are likely to have additional ingredients which would complicate the test. Mature corn is tested as corn meal mush with corn syrup, oats as oatmeal. With these, as with any food being tested, if there is no reaction within an hour then a second smaller portion is eaten.

Milk is taken as a large glass of milk, followed if there is no reaction with another glass an hour later. Eggs should be poached or soft boiled. Different varieties of cheese should be tested separately because reactions to them may be different and a response to different micro-organisms and not the milk from which the cheese was made. Cheddar cheese differs from other types. Cottage cheese should be dry and not the creamed variety.

Testing of other foods proceeds in a like manner—eggs, beef, peas, potato or whatever seems a likely possibility given your diet. Testing one food a day and undoubtedly missing some days because of social activities, having symptoms which would interfere with the interpretation of a test, and needing to abstain from a food for four days before testing and to have eaten it within 12 days can mean that a survey of your common foods can take several weeks, but at the end of that time you should have established clearly what your food allergens are. The thing to be most careful about is to be sure you are completely avoiding the test food for the four days before the test.

What kind of reactions will the test produce? This is highly variable for different individuals. Look for any changes that take place for the hour or two after eating. Check your pulse 30 and 60 minutes after eating to see if it rises abnormally. Does your nose feel different, either more stuffy or runny? How about your mouth and throat? Do you have a feeling of mucus in your throat or is there coughing? Does your skin feel cold or flushed? How about your stomach? Do you feel sick or queasy? Are there cramps or gas? Are there any different sensations in your arms or legs? Do you feel excited, irritable, depressed, listless, or sleepy? Do you have a headache? Is your vision affected? Is there sweating?

There probably will not be uncertainty as to whether a reaction has been produced. RRZ state that the reaction is "usually of such very definite nature that there is little doubt in the mind of either the patient or the physician that one is dealing with a specific cause and effect relationship."[37]

One may wonder, why should I go out of my way to deliberately try to provoke some unpleasant feelings? Why should I go out looking for a headache or an upset stomach or a coughing spell or whatever? The only reason can be the relief to be gained in the long run from detecting the foods which have been spoiling your life for you. The stronger and more unpleasant the reaction that you get, the more of a poison that food is for you and the better off you are in learning about it so you can avoid it.

Dr. Randolph discovered many years ago that, if an unpleasant reaction to a food does develop, it usually is associated with an increase in body acidity and can generally be relieved with an alkalizer. A teaspoon of sodium bicarbonate (ordinary baking soda) in an eight-ounce glass followed by a second glass of water will ordinarily help.[38] More effective is a mixture of two parts sodium bicarbonate to one part of potassium bicarbonate. The latter can be bought at a pharmacy or chemical supply dealer. A close approximation to this mixture is available as Alka-Seltzer "Special Antacid Formula" packaged in a gold-colored box. Regular Alka-Seltzer in the blue box contains aspirin which could be allergenic for some people and so should be avoided in this situation. A somewhat more extreme alternative is a teaspoon of magnesium sulphate (epsom salts) mixed well in a glass of warm water.[39] This not only acts as an alkalizer but helps to get the food out of the system quickly. An equivalent to this would be two ounces (two tablespoonsfull) of unflavored milk of magnesia.[40]

The effectiveness of alkalizers in dealing with known allergic reactions and their heavy use in our society makes one wonder whether many of the instances of headache, indigestion, gas, etc. for which these products are advertised and used are not really due to unsuspected allergy.

Sometimes a reaction may be delayed for several hours or even into the middle of the night or, as we have seen, the next morning. Even so, if one has been testing, the source of the reaction will be evident. Any food eaten after the test meal that day should be something which is known to be innocent or which was eaten the day preceding the test so as not to complicate the test interpretation. RRZ maintain that usually in the case of delayed reactions the person also has a reaction shortly after eating the food, but that it may be so mild that it is overlooked. An increased pulse after a test meal may signal a delayed reaction if there is no other response shortly after eating the test food.

After one's most frequently encountered allergens have been identified and eliminated from the diet, the same principles of testing may be applied to foods encountered in more ordinary circumstances. You find yourself feeling the way you did after testing a food which turned out to be allergenic, either shortly after eating or hours later. Knowing that your basic diet is innocent you can ask what you had to eat that was different. Very likely you will be able to quickly determine what the offending food was. If you wish to verify your suspicion, you can do so with a test of the food after four day's avoidance of it.

This then, is the essence of the deliberate food test. Any food which is questionable at any time can be tested with the method. A food which was found to be allergenic but which has been avoided for a period of time may be retested to see if sensitivity to it has been lost. In this case it need not have been eaten within 12 days of the test because the object is to find out if one is still sensitive to it from the last time it was eaten.

If it turns out on retest to be innocent, then it may be cautiously reintroduced into the diet as described earlier. Subsequent testing can show whether one remains insensitive to it. It may be, as happened in my case, that in the course of dropping some foods you eat others sufficiently often that you acquire a sensitivity to them. Any time one suspects this the questionable foods can be checked with this method.

RRZ had their patients do home testing, although usually after the patients had had one or more tests in the office. They found that home testing was "approximately 80% accurate."[41] Most inaccuracies were due to delayed reactions, situations where the person noted no symptoms within an hour after eating a food and concluded that it was not allergenic. Another way in which a delayed reaction could mislead would be if it showed up about the time the person ate the next meal, so the response would be attributed to the food just eaten rather than the test food. This is the reason any food eaten in a meal after the test should be a safe food which had been eaten the day or so preceding the test.

If a person is careful and gives full consideration to the possibility of delayed reactions, the accuracy rate should approach 100%. A recent book on clinical ecology stated: "Carried out under controlled conditions, the individual food test can be an extremely accurate and valid test for the specific diagnosis of food reactivity."[42]

Some conventional textbooks on allergy have questioned the accuracy of food consumption tests because consistent confirmatory results were not obtained with blind follow-up studies. In such a study the food to be tested would be prepared as a semi-liquid by a dietician and administered to the patient through a tube running directly into the stomach. The patient thus does not know what food is being given. Where such studies have not confirmed allergies as determined earlier, the most likely explanation is that the investigator did not allow for masking and take precautions to be sure that the later testing was done with the patient in an unmasked state.

Both Mackarness and Randolph have reported success with blind testing in verifying food sensitivities. In a case described by Mackarness, neither the patient nor the nursing staff in the hospital knew which foods were given at a particular time, but the innocent and the allergenic ones were clearly detectable by all.[43]

Although as Randolph has noted, such checks are not routinely done—it is unnecessarily time-consuming for the doctor and certainly an unpleasant procedure for the patient—enough such verifications have been made to show that ordinary food consumption tests are quite accurate. Randolph has also tested the power of suggestion on patients by telling them that some other food was being administered than actually was the case. When an innocent food was given but the patient was told it was one known to be allergenic no reaction to the food developed and when an allergenic food was given but the patient was told it was a safe food a reaction followed. Such tests show that the patients are really responding to their allergies and not to suggestion.[44]

These studies indicate that if you do or do not have a reaction to a particular food it is very likely that your response will be determined by the actual degree of your sensitivity to the food and not by what you think about it or expect might happen. When testing it is very helpful to keep a food-activities-symptoms diary as described earlier. Then, if there is any question about a reaction being a delayed one from a food eaten earlier or from one eaten at the next meal, the diary will provide a record which can serve as a basis for further tests that will provide an answer. After another period of at least four days of abstinence from the questioned test food, it can be eaten again, but followed with a different food, considered safe, at the next meal. If a reaction again appears, this would be evidence that it is a delayed one from the test food. Keeping a diary can thus aid in tracking down the real offenders.

Terms like "offender," "tracking down," "guilty," etc. suggest the image of a detective stalking the criminal, which is a quite appropriate image of the process. There is harm being done to an innocent person by an unknown assailant the victim is trying to identify. It is a matter of being a detective, but one who knows the method of operation of the villain.

One possible source of inaccuracy could be failure to avoid an allergen completely. This would be most likely with widely used foods such as milk, egg or corn, which find their way into many prepared foods in sufficient quantities to maintain masking. Again, simple foods prepared at home from known raw materials are the best protection against this possibility. Just one exposure during the four-day avoidance period could be enough to sustain masking.

Care with the tests and honesty with oneself are important for test accuracy. One patient always ate peanuts while drinking bourbon and (wrongly) judged his reaction as being due to the peanuts, not wishing to question the bourbon!

It should be clear that what has been said here regarding testing applies to adults or older teenagers. Yet, allergies can of course affect children, producing either physical symptoms or behavior difficulties (as will be covered in the next chapter), and the need to determine a child's allergens may even arise shortly after birth. Small children will probably not have the perspective and the vocabulary to note and report on the more subtle symptoms that can be important in detecting allergens with sublingual or individual feeding tests as just described here. Also, fasting is not recommended for children. As there is no evidence that skin testing is more accurate for children than for adults, such tests would not be very helpful in determining food allergies.

We are left, then, with some combination of an elimination diet and uncommon foods test for infants and small children. Everything said about allergy-addiction applies to children also, so that the guilty foods are almost certainly those eaten every day or so and those which are favorite foods. These may then be eliminated from the diet in an uncommon foods test the same as with adults. Then, if an improvement has been noted, the regular foods can be introduced back into the diet one at a time at intervals of several days, with careful observation of any effects produced by each new food. As with adults, a diary could prove very helpful.

There are two concerns which are particularly relevant to children. One is the matter of maintaining adequate nutrition while on either a testing or a permanent diet, which omits important foods. While adequate nutrition is important to everyone, it is even more so for a growing child. Probably the two most important factors in the diet which should be given attention are calcium and protein. Milk is an excellent source of both and egg provides very high quality protein. If these two commonly allergenic foods are avoided, then their nutritional values should be compensated for in other ways. Chewable calcium tablets are available and could be used to provide calcium; the use of other protein sources such as meat or fish could be increased to maintain protein intake.

The other concern is with the possibility that the child's diet may be contaminated by foods obtained outside the home. If the child eats his lunch at school, the only way a diet can be maintained is for him to bring his lunch from home and have him understand he is not to eat anything else. If the children have treats in the classroom on special occasions, the mother can send something ahead of time for the teacher to keep and give to the child in place of an allergenic food the other children are eating. My wife does this for children in her first grade classroom. Also the child should be cautioned about snacks or meals at the homes of friends.

References

1. Sheldon, John M., M.D., Lovell, Robert G., M.D. and Mathews, Kenneth P., M.D., *A Manual of Clinical*

Allergy, W. B. Saunders Co., Philadelphia, 1967, p. 201.

2. Sherman, William B., M.D., *Hypersensitivity: Mechanisms and Management*, W. B. Saunders Co., Philadelphia, 1968, p. 155.

3. Feingold, Ben F., M.D., *Introduction to Clinical Allergy*, Charles C. Thomas, Springfield, Ill., 1973, p. 148.

4. Crozier, Wallace, M.D., "Elimination Diets," in Speer, Frederic, M.D., and Dockhorn, Robert J., *Allergy and Immunology in Childhood*, Charles C. Thomas, Springfield, Ill., 1973, p. 371.

5. Rinkel, Herbert J., M.D., Randolph, Theron G., M.D. and Zeller, Michael, M.D., *Food Allergy*, Charles C. Thomas, Springfield, Ill., 1951, p. 145.

6. ibid., p. 170. emphasis in the original.

7. Philpott, William H., M.D., "Ecologic, Orthomolecular, and Behavioral Contributions to Psychiatry," *Journal of Orthomolecular Psychiatry*, Vol. 3, No. 4, p. 357.

8. Sherman, op. cit., p. 163.

9. Dickey, Lawrence D., M.D., F.A.C.S., *Clinical Ecology*, Charles C. Thomas, Springfield, Ill., 1976, p. 29.

10. Coca, Arthur F., M.D., *The Pulse Test*, ARC Books, New York, 1959, p. 16.

11. ibid., p. 62.

12. Coca, Arthur F., M.D., *Familial Nonreaginic Food Allergy*, 2nd edit., Charles C. Thomas, Springfield, Ill., 1945.

13. Coca, *The Pulse Test*, p. 49.

14. see, for example, Feingold, op. cit., p. 148.

15. Coca, *The Pulse Test*, p. 11.

16. ibid., p. 37.

17. Vaughan, Warren T. M.D., *Practice of Allergy*, C.V. Mosby, St. Louis, 1939, p. 332.

18. Rinkel, Randolph, and Zeller, op. cit., p. 236–37.

19. Crozier, op. cit., p. 371.

20. see, for example, Philpott, William H., M.D., "Maladaptive Reactions to Frequently Used Foods and Commonly Met Chemicals as Precipitating Factors in Many Chronic Physical and Chronic Emotional Illnesses," in Williams, Roger J., Ph.D., and Kalita, Dwight, K., Ph.D., *A Physician's Handbook on Orthomolecular Medicine*, Pergamon Press, New York, 1977, p. 143. Philpott specifies the first five qualifications; I thought it appropriate to add the sixth one.

21. Dickey, op. cit., p. 400.

22. Randolph, Theron G., M.D., "Ecologic Orientation in Medicine: Comprehensive Environmental Control in Diagnosis and Therapy," in Williams and Kalita, op. cit., p. 127.

23. Mackarness, Richard, M.D., *Eating Dangerously*, Harcourt, Brace, Jovanovich, New York, 1976, p. 52.

24. Mandell, Marshall, M.D., "The Diagnostic Value of Therapeutic Fasting and Food Ingestion Tests in a Controlled Environment," *Journal International Academy Metabology*, Vol. IV, No. 1, March 1975, p. 79.

25. ibid., p. 80.

26. ibid., p. 81.

27. ibid., p. 79.

28. Philpott, op. cit., p. 143.

29. Mackarness, op. cit., pp. 129-30.

30. ibid., p. 130.

31. ibid., p. 134.

32. Rinkel, Randolph, and Zeller, op. cit., p. 125.

33. information on Drs. Mitchell and Hosen supplied by Dr. Marshall Mandell in a personal communication.

34. Dickey, op. cit., p. 400.

35. Philpott, William H., M.D., *Ecological Medicine Manual*, Oklahoma City, Oklahoma, 1975 (mimeographed), p. 29.

36. Rinkel, Randolph, and Zeller, op. cit., pp. 64-5.

37. ibid., p. 12.
38. Randolph, Theron G., M.D., "The Enzymatic, Acid, Hypoxia, Endocrine Concept of Allergic Inflammation," in Dickey, op. cit., p. 589. Mandell, Marshall, M.D., personal communication.
39. Mackarness, op. cit., p. 127.
40. Mandell, personal communication.
41. Rinkel, Randolph, and Zeller, op. cit., p. 215.
42. Dickey, op. cit., p. 400.
43. Mackarness, op. cit., p. 10.
44. Randolph, Theron G., M.D., "Ecologic Orientation in Medicine: Comprehensive Environmental Control in Diagnosis and Therapy," in Williams, Roger J., Ph.D. and Kalita, Dwight K., Ph.D., eds., *A Physician's Handbook on Orthomolecular Medicine*, Pergamon Press, New York, 1977, p. 127.

CHAPTER 6

Allergy and Behavioral Problems

MANY BOOKS ON allergy, including both those written for medical professionals and those addressed to the layman, are organized mainly according to symptoms. Thus, one might find chapters on asthma, skin allergies, etc. As we have seen, though, allergy can produce a great variety of symptoms, a number of them frequently being found in the same person. Accordingly, I have usually just spoken of sensitivity to a substance or of a reaction or response to an allergen, it being understood that practically any kind of physical symptom or condition may be due to allergy.

In this chapter I wish to be more specific, however, and look at some manifestations of allergy. I do this because some of these one may never think of as being attributable to allergy. While we saw that most conventional allergists are reluctant to believe that a whole host of symptoms may be due to allergy, at least it seems somewhat possible that various physical conditions can be allergically caused. That the realm of behavior could also be influenced by allergy appears so unlikely that it requires special consideration.

As a sociologist, I look for social determinants of behavior—family influences, peer group pressures, social status, group relationships, and the like—but I am committed to trying to understand human behavior however it may be influenced. Furthermore, if in trying to understand family relationships, for example, I find that they are affected by such physical factors as allergy, then this has indeed helped me to comprehend the family. What I am getting at is the effect allergy can have on human behavior. While such a topic may seem rather "far out," there is good evidence that some types of problem behavior are influenced by allergy and this is what the present chapter will concern itself with.

Children's Hyperactivity:
The Feingold Approach

Attracting increasing attention in the past decade or so is the phenomenon of children's restlessness and overactivity. The most common term used to refer to the condition is hyperactivity, although it has also been called hyperkinesis, minimal brain dysfunction (MBD), as well as a number of other terms. Not surprisingly, the problem has attracted the most attention in the schoolroom where the teacher finds that Johnny can't sit still or pay attention to his work long enough to learn anything. Such children have poor concentration, keep piping up at inopportune moments that disrupt the whole class, and generally are a problem to themselves, other children, teachers and administrators, and of course their parents and other family members. An old-fashioned teacher is likely to view the problem as a behavior deviation—the child is being naughty—and use punishment. Most modern teachers have come to think of it as a medical condition and suggest that the child see a doctor. Indeed, in innumerable cases parents have been told by school officials that the child *must* be given medication by a doctor in order to be permitted to continue attending school. From the standpoint of clinical ecology, both approaches are wrong.

Let us take a look at just what hyperactivity can involve in individual cases. One mother described her life as "a living hell" which began when she brought her boy home from the hospital. He slept so little and screamed so much that the neighbors thought the parents were regularly beating him. The parents "were constantly at each other's throats" over trouble stemming from their son, they could neither entertain relatives at home nor go out themselves because no one would do the babysitting.

The mother still has scars from attacks on her by the boy, but the father has recovered from a broken hand he suffered when frustration led him to smash his fist against the wall. In kindergarten the boy threw temper tantrums and tried to strangle other children. Before the boy's behavior became normal as a result of treating it as allergy-caused, the family had spent $75,000 on medical and other expenses.[1] They were not as fortunate as the family that wound up spending only $30,000 on their child.[2]

While all cases are not as extreme as this, there is little doubt but that a hyperactive child is a very disruptive influence in family, school and community. There is no way life can be normal for brothers or sisters of such a problem child. A hyperactive child affects many others.

The child taken to a doctor and diagnosed as hyperactive is in an unusual medical situation. There are no x-rays or laboratory tests that can suggest or confirm a diagnosis, so despite an imposing name for the condition like minimal brain dysfunction, the evidence really comes from reports of parents or teachers that the child is restless and unruly. Curiously, for children the thing that seems to calm them down is not a tranquilizer or barbituate, but an "upper," an amphetamine of the type that makes adults more alert and active. The most commonly prescribed such drug for hyperactivity is a product called Ritalin. In

Omaha a few years ago it was found that one child out of seven was on the stuff. One school district in California had 30%—almost one child in three![3]

Estimates in the early 1970's placed somewhere between 250,000 and 300,000 children in America as users of Ritalin, with 243 million Ritalin tablets being sold, half of them for hyperkinesis.[4] A number of other drugs are also prescribed in lesser quantities for this condition. Side effects of the stimulant type drugs such as Ritalin are less serious than for tranquilizers, but still include nervousness, insomnia, stomach ache and skin rash.[5] This, then, has been the answer of conventional medicine to the problem of the child who cannot behave normally in the classroom.

If the treatment were completely safe and effective, there would be little reason to question it, but there are serious doubts on both issues. Ritalin does not calm down all children and many remain about as disruptive as they were before. The difference is that the teacher now thinks that nothing more can be done and so does not press for further action. Potentially much more serious is the fact that nobody knows what the long-range effects are on a growing child of regular administration of a drug that alters the functioning of its nervous system. Will it be found eventually, as has been done with a number of other drugs, that harm has been done which only becomes evident years later?

It might appear to some people that the hyperactive behavior of today's children is simply a response to the strain and complexity of modern life—international tensions reported daily, crowded cities, social unrest, etc.—except that other urban-industrial nations such as those in western Europe which have similar conditions do not have a children's hyperkinesis problem. In England, for example, hyperactivity is found in only one child in 2,000.[6]

It was an allergist, specifically Dr. Ben F. Feingold, chief (now emeritus) of the Allergy Clinic of the Kaiser-Permanente Medical Center at San Francisco, who found an answer within the field of allergy to a substantial part of the hyperactivity problem. Dr. Feingold speaks of H-LD/MBD (hyperkinesis-learning disability/minimal brain dysfunction) children and notes that not all will be overactive. Some simply have a muscle coordination problem. "The child cannot easily button a coat, or if older, tie shoe laces or participate successfully in sports."[7] If hand incoordination is combined with eye disturbances, then difficulties in reading and writing are highly likely. These in turn will lead to relative failure in the classroom, which can result in the child being stigmatized both by its peers and the teacher. Behavior problems would be a likely consequence, but in such cases would be an indirect result of H-LD/MBD.

After more than 20 years of private practice, Dr. Feingold joined Kaiser-Permanente as chief of the Department of Allergy in 1951. He became interested in the question of aspirin-sensitivity in patients with allergies. Aspirin is not infrequently a source of trouble for those with allergies (I was advised not to use aspirin by an allergist). A potentially sensitive person may take it repeatedly with no trouble, but then quickly develop a sensitivity so severe that it actually threatens life. A reaction such as shortness of breath after taking aspirin should be a warning to avoid it absolutely in the future.

Chemically, aspirin is called a salicylate, a substance which also is found naturally in some foods. In managing aspirin-sensitive patients, Dr. Feingold had them avoid not just aspirin but all foods containing salicylates, which includes almonds, apples, apricots, the more commonly used berries, cherries, currants, grapes and raisins, nectarines, oranges, peaches, and plums and prunes.[8] Then he learned that other substances could evoke symptoms in aspirin-sensitive persons. Two London researchers demonstrated that a medication distinctly different from aspirin chemically, nevertheless, worked within the body the same way as aspirin does.

Theorizing that other substances used in artificial food flavorings and colorings could do this also, Dr. Feingold modified his diet for aspirin-sensitive patients so that it excluded not only all foods containing salicylates but all foods and drugs with artificial colorings or flavorings. "From that point on," he wrote, "we were overwhelmingly successful in patient management."[9] It was this diet that was given to the $75,000 boy described above. Within two days of starting it, he slept normally for the first time in his life. After "a few months there was an absolutely unbelievable difference. Now he's a normal child."[10]

At the time Dr. Feingold developed his aspirin-sensitive diet, which was the mid-1960's, he had no particular interest in problems of behavior or even any knowledge of the "critical situation in hyperkinesis and learning disability that was developing throughout the country."[11] However, in using his diet to clear up physical symptoms such as hives he found that patients, both child and adult, not uncommonly had behavioral problems alleviated also. One woman who was described as hostile and aggressive and who was having serious problems both at home and at work was near the end of her second year of unsuccessful psychotherapy. Within 10 days after beginning the salicylate-free diet, her behavior became normal, which so surprised her psychiatrist that he called Dr. Feingold to ask what he had done. Public concern with the hyperactivity problem by the early 1970's helped to focus Feingold's interest on the problem, leading him to write the book, *Why Your Child Is Hyperactive*.

Why should hyperactivity have become such a problem? Dr. Feingold points to the tremendous increase in the use of artificial colorings and flavorings since World War II. While most people can consume them without difficulty, some are sensitive to them and respond with abnormal aggressive or hyperactive behavior. While technically Dr. Feingold does not consider such responses to be true allergy, for all practical purposes they might just as well be. They result from consuming substances by people who are sensitive to them.

Consider the situation prior to World War II. About two-thirds of the breakfast cereal sold was hot cereal, practically all of which was simply processed natural grains. Now the greatest part of cereals are highly processed cold cereals, the vast majority with artificial colorings or flavorings or both. While artificial colorings and flavorings have been around during all of the 20th century, the extent of their use has exploded in the past few decades. There is hardly a processed food which does not contain one or the other or both—meats, including self-basting turkeys; puddings; baked goods; ice cream and other frozen confections; candy; soft drinks; even dog food! While traveling one time, I got a hamburger at a franchise of one of the national fast-food chains and was surprised to find that the bun was yellow. At one time that would have meant eggs in the dough. In this case I am sure it meant artificial coloring. A person getting the hamburger, a milk shake, and pie would get loaded with additives. Even a white frosting may have artificial coloring to make it a particular *kind* of white.

As a doctor, Feingold is seriously concerned about artificial colorings and flavorings in medicines, which people these days want to look and taste good. For the sensitive person an additive-loaded medication could produce a worse problem than the condition it is intended to help. No one knows how many synthetic flavors are used in America. It seems certain it is over a thousand. Why are not more European children hyperactive? France permits only seven synthetic flavors, which certainly must be part of the answer.[12]

What happens when the hyperactive child grows up? Is the condition outgrown? What we have seen about allergies in general not being outgrown should make us cautious here. Because hyperactivity has been recognized as a medical problem only so recently, there is no reservoir of cases who were diagnosed as having the condition 20 or 30 years ago and who could now be studied to see how they fare as middle-aged adults. Because of lesser use of additives in earlier decades, the causes of hyperactivity were not as prevalent.

One factor which could make it seem that hyperactivity is not carried into adult life is that, by age 18, the person is no longer required by law to be confined to a classroom where he is expected to concentrate and be quiet. In adult life the person can find a job and lifestyle in which his restlessness and short attention span are not of serious social consequence. We can wonder whether some social deviates—people who cannot hold a job, who get into fights and social scrapes regularly and are difficult to live with, and perhaps who are even legal offenders—have allergy as a contributing cause. Dr. Feingold, while recognizing that adolescence can bring about changes which ease the condition for some children, nevertheless, believes one should not expect the condition to correct itself and that even if it would "there may be psychological hangovers from years of battling within and without."[13] He also quotes from a letter sent him by someone with first-hand experience who wrote: "We hyperkinetic children do become hyperkinetic adults. I should know. I am 35 years old and still suffer."

Dr. Feingold does not claim that every case of hyperactivity can be corrected with the K-P (Kaiser-

Permanente) Diet, which eliminates both foods containing natural salicylates and foods with artificial colorings and flavorings. For some children the issue is also complicated by their having allergies in addition to salicylate-additive sensitivities. Overall, Feingold estimates that half the H-LD children respond completely to the K-P Diet, while an additional 25% improve enough to no longer need medication.[14]

A letter from a parent in *Prevention* magazine (January 1978, p. 166) describes another type of condition that was aided by the Feingold diet. A two-year-old boy was not really hyperactive but just "very unhappy." He "slept very little, cried a lot, hung on Mommy and found it difficult to settle down once he would get upset." He was very nice at times, however. The child's pediatrician recommended the Feingold diet, and on it the child soon became "a normal, happy little boy."

Problems arising from trying to follow the diet can result either from the difficulties in trying to identify and obtain additive-free foods or from alterations it may necessitate in patterns of living. As a means of dealing with the first issue, Dr. Feingold has proposed a logo for use on the labels of food products that do not contain any chemical additives. (See Fig. 1, page 129).

The second problem, interference with present-day lifestyles, can be a serious one for some families. They have to combat television commercials, particularly on children's programs, which constantly push the consumption of additive-loaded goodies. The child has to learn to pass up the sociability associated with a candy bar or glass of fruit punch urged on him at an after-school stop at the home of well-intentioned but uncomprehending friends. The child's parents find that breakfast can no longer be a toasted tart or a bowl of colored crunchies and a glass of fruit drink; an afternoon snack of a doughnut and a soft drink are out. Suppers can not be simple factory-made items from a can or the freezer. Even meat extender preparations for homemade dishes are excluded.

Many parents seem unable to really follow the diet rigidly, which is what is required for its success. The diaries of some families who were not successful showed repeated lapses, 17 within 14 days for one family. As one exposure can affect a child for more than a day, this amounts to no control at all. Another family which was being torn apart by the behavior of its eight-year-old to the point of needing counseling, still thought that the diet would be "too much for them."[15] One mother, interviewed on a television program, was unwilling to try the Feingold approach because: "I'm not a kitchen type of person." In some cases children have refused to follow the diet, even though they have a strong aversion to the pills they would get otherwise.

Thus we find ourselves in the position of having a means which is frequently effective in dealing with a problem, but with some people not being willing to make the behavioral changes needed to employ that means. At least we know, however, what the situation is. We would probably all be better off if fewer additives were in our food supply. Our government is much more lenient in this regard than most other countries, due mainly to political pressures from the companies that profit from making or using additives. If these can not be eliminated at least they should be identified on the label so that people can know what they are buying and consuming.

Within two years of the publication of Dr. Feingold's book, mothers of hyperactive children had organized some 80 chapters of the Feingold Association, with the Philadelphia chapter having some 650 members and the Houston chapter including over 100 doctors.[16] A national headquarters office has been established (Drawer AG, Holtsville, N.Y., 11742) which publishes a newsletter and

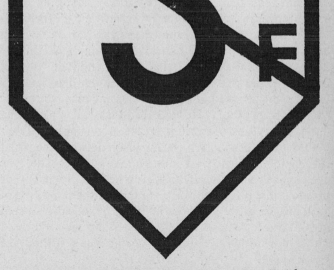

Fig. 1 Feingold Logo for Additive-Free Foods

provides information on additives and hyperactivity. The New York chapter claims that eliminating preservatives from the diet as well as artificial colorings and flavorings results in an even higher rate of success than has been obtained with the original Feingold K-P diet.[17]

While visiting Dr. Mandell's clinic, I got a vivid view of the effect of a food additive on a person sensitive to it. Without knowing what she was being tested for, a woman being given some extract sublingually became depressed, started to tremble, and even to cry soon after receiving it. The extract turned out to be a yellow food coloring solution. Given a turnoff relieving dose, she quickly returned to normal, but there was no question but that the food color solution had a strong effect upon her.

At the time he wrote *Why Your Child Is Hyperactive*, Dr. Feingold placed almost complete emphasis upon artificial food colorings and flavorings. The only other additive he mentioned was the preservative, BHT (Butylated Hydroxy Toluene), and then only to state: "An occasional child may show an adverse reaction to BHT."[18] Since then he has found that many children "do not respond to the diet until BHT has been omitted—and it's found in breakfast foods, cooking fats and oils, even butter and oleomargarine."[19] He has called for BHT to be phased out and eventually banned from the food supply. All that is needed is a distribution system which does not keep food sitting indefinitely in warehouses and on shelves. There is a question as to whether BHT is even needed. Some brands of foods contain it while other brands of the same kind of food do just as well without it. While practically all cold breakfast cereals now contain BHT, cold cereals were sold successfully for decades prior to World War II without the preservative.

Vending machines and lunchrooms in schools themselves are frequently contributors to the food additive problem. The increasingly common school hot lunch programs are likely to contain additive-loaded dishes. The menu at the school where my wife teaches regularly has an item whose flavor is so indeterminate that it is described only as "red jello." On other days fruit flavored frozen confections with catchy Madison Avenue names are featured. Hot dogs, pizzas and sloppy Joe's are popular with children and can be made without additives but this requires the knowledge and attention of those responsible for preparing the foods. In my wife's school, as in many others, the items are not prepared locally but have been commercially produced and are simply heated up at the site. With school breakfast programs also becoming more widespread, the chances for additives is further increased.

Artificially colored and flavored high-sugar confections are big sellers for vending machines. In various communities around the country people concerned with health issues have sought to have these items removed but have usually been met with the argument from school officials that these machines produce much revenue which helps to support school programs. But vending machines can also dispense healthful products and concerned citizens have been effective in a number of places in getting natural food items placed in vending machines. One particularly successful parents' group is in Greenburgh Central School District in Westchester County, New York. Its efforts even resulted in a large national baking concern changing its recipes so as to use natural rather than artificial colors.[20]

Although his approach touches on clinical ecology, Dr. Feingold would not be considered to be a clinical ecologist by others in the field, and there is no evidence that he considers himself to be one. Rather, he is a conventional allergist who developed a particular theory about allergy and behavior. But while labels are not important in themselves, they can indicate ways of thinking.

Clinical ecologists appreciate that he has focused more attention on the effects environmental substances can have upon behavior, but as described by Dr. Marshall Mandell, Feingold's ideas on the subject are both limited and limiting.[21] By placing emphasis just upon salicylates, Feingold overlooks other substances, both food and chemical, in the child's environment that can also influence behavior (we will consider chemical allergens in the next chapter). We have seen that the salicylate-free K-P diet "cures" only about half the hyperactive children and aids to some extent another one-fourth. This is not exactly complete success. Dr. Mandell asks, if it is just a matter of salicylates, why children have not been made hyperactive by naturally-occurring salicylates in such foods as apples, cherries, etc. which have been around all the time?

There is a likely clue in the fact noted earlier that the success rate for the K-P diet was higher when preservatives and BHT were also excluded. The lesson from this, and one which is elementary to clinical ecologists, is that we need to look at the total environment of the person, not just to a few specific substances, whether natural foods or chemicals. Artificial food colors are made from coal-tar, a substance classified as a chemical hydrocarbon. We will have more to say about hydrocarbons later; it will suffice here to note that there are many other chemical compounds in the hydrocarbon family and that any of them can severely affect both the physical and mental functioning of individuals. Any food additive, including the numerous hydrocarbons, can affect susceptible people, and the fewer of them there are in the diet the less trouble they will cause.

In calling for elimination of artificial colorings and flavorings, the K-P diet brings about a considerable change in the kind of foods which the child eats. A much smaller proportion of its food can be bought ready-prepared, so that there is also a considerable decrease in the overall load of chemical additives that the child is exposed to, besides the decrease in colorings and flavorings. If foods containing BHT and other preservatives are also ruled out, this further eliminates another group of foods also containing chemical additives—practically all cold breakfast cereals, for example, as well as instant mashed potatoes, prepared meat-extender concoctions, etc. The family is forced into having simple foods prepared from scratch. Thus, the success of the K-P diet in many cases may come about not from the reduction in salicylates but from the reduced exposure to other chemicals that it incidentally brings about.

While the K-P diet concerns itself with just one segment of the overall environment impinging upon the child, clinical ecology concerns itself with the whole range of possible trouble-causing substances. While there seems to be no question but that the K-P diet has produced some stunning successes, it also has a failure rate that would not be tolerated by clinical ecologists. The biggest danger to the Feingold approach, as viewed by Dr. Mandell, is that it so frequently doesn't work, and that its failures can lead parents to give up the search for something in the environment that is producing the problem behavior. If the K-P diet fails in a particular case, it may not mean that the child doesn't have an environmentally-caused problem, only that the diet concerns itself with only one aspect of the total situation, and one which is not relevant for that particular child. It is not that the Feingold approach is wrong, but that from the standpoint of clinical ecology it is just incomplete.

Allergy and Children's Behavior Problems

Certainly there is evidence that many other substances, both food and chemical, can cause children's behavior problems. Psychologist K. E. Moyer quotes from the letter of a mother who reported that within 20 minutes of eating banana her small boy would have a temper tantrum. He also was allergic to all types of sugar except maple sugar.[22]

In another case described by Professor Moyer, a five-year-old boy was too uncontrollable to take an I.Q. test. His speech development was so poor that it was believed he suffered from aphasia. His EEG (brain wave test) showed definite abnormalities. Allergy testing revealed him to be sensitive to milk, chocolate and cola, all of which were eliminated from his diet. Seven and a half months later another test showed his EEG to be normal and behavior was much improved. When given the allergenic foods for a week, he again became uncontrollable and his EEG once more showed abnormalities.

For the sake of society as well as the individual, we need, as Moyer stated, a safe and effective means for the control of violence. Certainly allergy should be considered.

Other doctors confirm that allergy, whether to additives or to foods themselves, can affect many children. Dr. Lendon H. Smith, while conceding that "the Feingold idea is very valid,"[23] reports that he has had more success eliminating sugar and white flour from problem children's diets. These simple carbohydrates can have a profound effect upon some people, as will be discussed in a later chapter. The small child of a colleague of mine goes into a flurry of hyperactivity every time after having anything containing sugar, which is ordinarily kept out of his diet. When he is sick, however, and needs medication which they cannot get without sugar, his parents face the choice between withholding medication and putting up with a period of supercharged behavior.

Dr. Allan Cott has also found sugar to be a major cause of children's behavior problems. He has said: "The first thing I do with a hyperactive child is remove all soft drinks, cake, cookies, candy, ice-cream and sugared cereals from his diet. In nearly every instance, the child is markedly calmer within a very short time."[24] Dr. Cott realizes the difficulties in getting a nine- or 10-year-old child to abstain completely from candy, soft drinks and other junk foods loaded with sugar and white flour, but has devised a way to help the child come to understand the effects these foods can have upon him or her.

In cooperation with the parents, he asks if the child will agree to abstain from all junk foods for six days, if he or she can have all the junk foods desired on the seventh day. Most children will agree readily and really follow their diet during the six days. Ordinarily Saturday is the junk food day, when the child can have whatever it wants. Sunday is then miserable and Monday produces a terrible day at school. There is gradual improvement during the week so that by Friday the child feels good and things are going well. Then the next day of junk food starts the cycle all over again. A few weeks of this reveal very clearly to children the effects junk foods have upon them, so that they realize for themselves they should avoid these things and not see the restrictions as something arbitrarily imposed from the outside. As Dr. Cott says about this approach: "In so many cases the child is able to exercise the judgment that these things make him feel bad...."[25]

Of course, eliminating sugar and white flour from the diet also eliminates most bakery products and many other prepared foods, all of which tend to be loaded with additives. Nevertheless, while there seems little doubt but that many of these additives can make some children hyperactive, the role of allergy to foods themselves as a cause of behavior problems cannot be overlooked. Although Dr. Smith has found sugar and white flour to be particularly common allergens for children, he has also traced problems back to milk, cereal, chocolate, etc.

Similarly, pediatrician William G. Crook has emphasized the role of sugar as a culprit but has likewise noted that allergy to other foods can cause behavior problems in children. In a letter in *Pediatrics*, he recommends that doctors test for allergy by a "carefully planned elimination diet" before prescribing drugs such as Ritalin.

Just as with adults, allergy can be responsible for a whole host of other children's conditions, according to Dr. Crook.[26] Some of these are the same as for adults while others seem to be more characteristic of children. Bedwetting and false anemia—pale complexion with circles under the eyes—are examples of the latter. Learning problems, which may or may not be associated with hyperactivity, is another difficulty which Dr. Crook has found amenable to elimination of allergic foods from the child's diet. It is not surprising that Dr. Crook gets his leads as to which foods are most likely to be troublemakers by asking what are the child's favorites. These foods are usually the guilty ones, and improvement ordinarily follows when these are eliminated from the diet.

Parents of problem children could get some helpful insights and recommendations from Dr. Lendon Smith's book, *Improving Your Child's Behavior Chemistry* (Prentice-Hall, 1976, or Pocket Books). Dr. Smith believes that much children's problem behavior results not from bad parenting but from the inborn makeup of the child as it encounters certain environmental situations. Even if inborn characteristics are important in determining the child's behavior, this does not mean that nothing can be done, because, of course, the other side of the coin is the child's environment.

Dr. Smith points out that problem children can deviate in two ways—either they can be withdrawn and underactive or else too outgoing and overactive. The first type he calls the "withdrawers" and the second the "approachers."

Even the withdrawers, he says, can become passive because of such factors as too much stimuli impinging upon them (sensory overload) or from dietary imbalances. But except in extreme cases of pathological withdrawal, they tend not to attract attention as problem cases. The approachers, on the other hand, respond to overstimulation with excess physical activity and hence quickly get noticed. Dr. Smith points out that approachers are not likely to become doctors because their need for activity conflicts with the "long boring lectures" which are part of medical education.[27] Hence doctors have a hard time understanding the hyperactive individuals, whose personalities are so different from those of their own.

Dr. Smith has observed that behavior problem children tend to come from families having a history of such conditions as obesity, diabetes, hypoglycemia, alcoholism, allergies, migraine, insomnia and mental illness. This combination of conditions can seem quite natural to a clinical ecologist. Dr. Smith also comments: "It has been known for a long time that allergic people are susceptible to infections. The phlegm in the nasal and bronchial passages from milk, dust, mold or other inhalants is a good medium for bacterial growth. Sinusitis sufferers usually end up in the allergists' offices. Allergic children are more prone to ear, respiratory, intestinal, urinary, and skin infections. They have more than their share of virus infections and high fevers."[28]

Although he apparently does not test for foods systematically, Dr. Smith has found, as have others, that the most likely problem causers are milk, wheat, eggs, and sugar, which he recommends dropping from the diet of children who tend to have frequent illnesses.

While recognizing the frequent contribution that allergy makes both to physical illness and to behavior difficulties, Dr. Smith does not give much evidence in his book of using clinical ecology techniques or principles in detecting allergens. Nevertheless, many of his recommendations regarding diet and nutrition are in accord with what is described here. Supplemented with a clinical ecology viewpoint, Dr. Smith's book would be a valuable one for any parent.

Visual Evidence of
Behavior Change
from Allergy

People's minute-to-minute behavior is not the sort of thing that one can get down on paper and present in a book. Social scientists frequently use standardized systems for recording observations made of people's behavior by trained observers for research purposes, but these are descriptions of behavior rather than the concrete results of it. One way to obtain the latter, which has been employed by Dr. Marshall Mandell, is to obtain samples of the person's handwriting or other paper-and-pencil activity, both when he or she is "normal" and when reacting to an allergenic substance. Paper-and-pencil activity reflects thinking processes, emotions, perception and motor coordination, so that it is a sensitive indicator of overall functioning. I am grateful to Dr. Mandell for permitting me to present the examples given here. This material shows how some people can have their behavior affected by allergic reactions.

Fig. 2 through Fig. 5 are handwriting samples of a 10-year-old girl with hay fever and asthma as well as headaches, nausea, dizziness, erratic school performance and episodes of bizarre behavior.

Fig. 6 through Fig. 8 show the handwriting of an eight-year-old boy with periods of both overactivity and underactivity, memory impairment and inability to con-

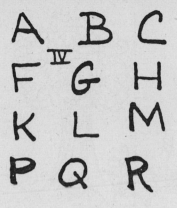

Fig. 2. Portion of alphabet made when not reacting to an allergenic substance.

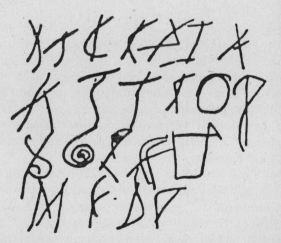

Fig. 3. Alphabet made when given provocative test for chemical hydrocarbons.

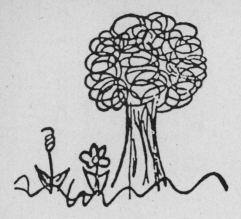

Fig. 4. Drawing of a tree made when not reacting to an allergenic substance.

centrate.

Also during wheat test (Fig. 8), he was asked to write numbers from 1 to 5. Wrote "4, 3, 2," instead, then marked over them when realized he had not done it right.

His reactions were similar to those for wheat when tested with egg, chemical hydrocarbon, cane sugar and food preservatives. When asked to print his name while being tested for milk, he was unable to do so because he could not remember how to spell it.

Fig. 9 and Fig. 10 are samples of the handwriting of an adult female with a number of physical symptoms.

In addition to penmanship changes, this patient experienced burning throat, coughing, headache, post-nasal drip, nausea, shoulder and neck muscle spasms, loss of hand and arm strength, forearm muscle ache, chills, pressure in temples, and brief loss of contact with surroundings.

Mental Illness

Can allergy affect people in a way that produces mental and behavioral problems other than hyperactivity? A growing group of doctors is coming to the conclusion that the answer definitely is yes. A number of psychiatrists has been led to study allergy as a cause of even serious mental illness and much of the work in the clinical ecology approach to allergy has been done by psychiatrists with this orientation. Some of them have already been mentioned as important contributors to the understanding of allergy.

Randolph, although not a psychiatrist, found back in the 1940s that allergy could alter mental functioning. One patient, too confused to be permitted to be safely on her own in the city, was hospitalized for allergy testing. She had routinely drunk large amounts of coffee with beet sugar.

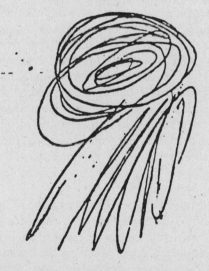

Fig. 5. Tree drawing when given provocative test for chemical hydrocarbons.

After having beets for supper she became very psychotic, Dr. Randolph recalled: "This was inconceivable. At 6:00 she was fine, but at 8:30 she was psychotic. . . . When I saw her the next morning she didn't know who she was, where she was, who I was. She was completely out of contact with her surroundings."[29] It took her two and a half days to return to normality. When she was given food through a tube so that she did not know what she was getting, beets produced the same reaction. It was the first case Randolph observed of a severe psychotic reaction to allergenic foods but he says that since then he has seen "thousands of cases."

Mackarness treated a women in England who had been admitted to a mental hospital 13 times for depression and violent behavior. She would slash her forearms, not necessarily in an attempt to commit suicide but simply as an expression of extreme tension. She had knocked unconscious her three-and-a-half-year-old son and thrown an older daughter out of the house right through a closed window. After having tried all conventional treatments, most doctors were ready to perform a lobotomy—a surgical procedure on the brain which usually makes the person more manageable but at the expense of having a dull almost zombie-like personality. Under Mackarness' direction she tried food tests and a number of allergenic foods were discovered. As a result of avoiding them in her diet, her personality changed completely; she became happy, was able to work outside, and became a good mother and housekeeper.[90]

A patient described in one paper is sensitive to sugar and wheat and "suffers from chronic schizophrenia which is rather easily controlled unless he ignores his prescribed diet."[31] After eating a piece of apple pie "he began actively hallucinating, was quite delusional and angry, and uncontrollable."[32] Mandell reported on a brilliant but violently schizophrenic man who had been ill many years,

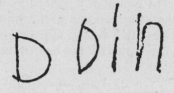

Fig. 6. Name printed with normal penmanship.

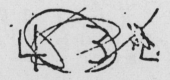

Fig. 7. Printing when undergoing provocative test for wheat. Note repeated "D", omitted "A" and "R", lower case "i" and "n".

![Fig. 8]

Fig. 8

and was dangerous to his family when at home. After a five-day fast "our patient was almost miraculously restored to a normal state of mental health. A truly beautiful, clear thinking person emerged from what had been a chaotic and at times treacherous animal-like being."[33]

Randolph coined the term ecological mental illness to refer to mental abnormalities produced by exposure to foods or chemicals to which the person was sensitive. Mandell later showed that it also applied to children and added the concept of infantile ecological mental illness. It is very easy to show that ecological mental illness is due to sensitivity to food and/or chemicals by using the basic technique developed by Rinkle and Randolph of having the patient avoid allergy-addictive substances for from four to 12 days and then re-exposing him to those substances one at a time. Doing so "has demonstrated the emergence of every shade of symptom described as schizophrenic, neurotic, or character neurotic plus a host of common somatic symptoms often dubbed as psychosomatic."[34] On the basis of statistics plus his own experience, Philpott has

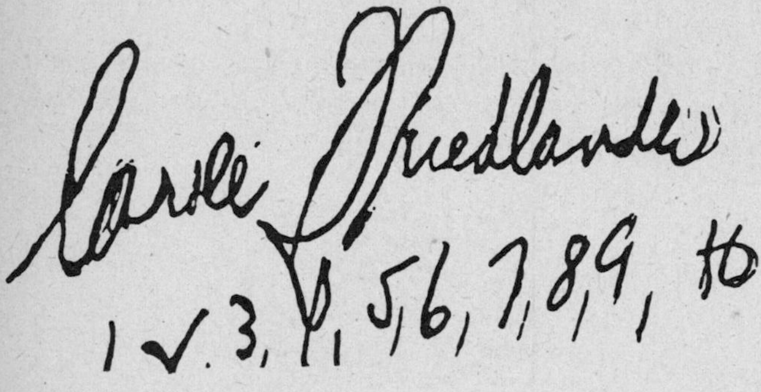

Fig. 9. Normal penmanship.

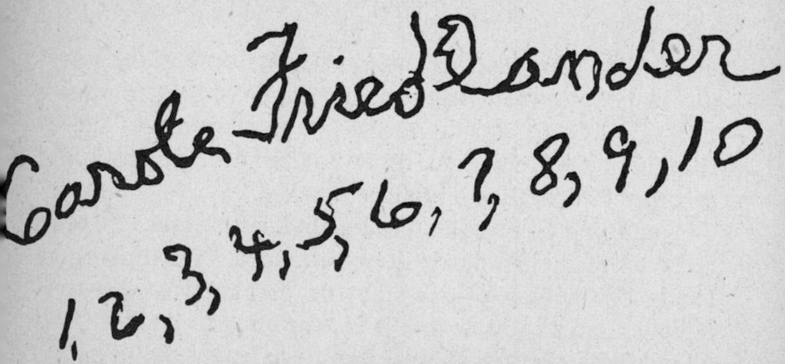

Fig. 10. Penmanship during tobacco smoke test.

concluded that an allergy-addictive state "can be demonstrated to exist niney-two per cent of the time in schizophrenia and likely exists in all schizophrenics."[35]

Randolph and Mandell have both made movies of psychotic states induced by substances to which the individuals are sensitive and have shown them to international conferences. Psychiatrists in other countries seem more interested in these findings than American psychiatrists. While Dr. Randolph has gotten a welcome reception at numerous international psychiatric congresses in other parts of the world, both the American Medical Association and the American Psychiatric Association resisted him or any other clinical ecologist give a presentation at their meetings,[36] following the typical pattern of rejecting information before finding out what it was. The American Psychiatric Association finally agreed to permit a session on allergy and behavior in its 1979 annual meeting in Chicago, with panel participants including Drs. Randolph, Mandell, and Philpott, as well as others who have been actively practising clinical ecology but who have not written as extensively on it. While this indication of acceptance of clinical ecology and the idea of ecological mental illness by conventional medicine is heartening, it was far too long delayed.

The most likely explanation for ecological mental illness is that of cerebral allergy. We know that different people respond to an allergen in different ways with different parts of the body being affected; one person breaks out in hives, another produces excess nasal mucus, while still another develops intestinal problems, etc. Given that practically any part of the body can be affected by an allergen, it would be strange if the brain and central nervous system of some people did not prove to be the vulnerable part for some people. Thus, just as allergy can produce tissue changes in the skin or mucous passages which are clearly evident, so could it lead to fluid secretion, swelling, changes in circulation, etc. which would affect the brain. Fluid secretions and swelling of surrounding tissues could increase pressure on the brain and biochemical changes related to the allergic reaction could alter the brain chemistry. While these things would not be visible from the outside, they could alter mental functioning and produce psychotic or neurotic behavior.[37]

At a conference recently, another ecologically oriented psychiatrist, Dr. H. L. Newbold, expressed doubt that the possible effects of tissue irritation itself as a cause of altered behavior. Nevertheless, while the exact mechanism by which psychotic behavior is produced by allergens is yet to be agreed upon, there is much evidence to show that many patients can have their behavior abnormalities turned "on" or "off" by the foods they eat.

Based on reports of success from Russia, Dr. Allan Cott has been investigating controlled fasting as a treatment for schizophrenia.[38] The method requires the cooperation of the patient and so cannot be imposed on an unwilling subject. Following the fast, which may last for three weeks or more, the patient is put on a controlled diet. The patient is carefully monitored for physiological functioning during the process. Only very difficult cases were selected by Cott for treatment with this method. "A prerequisite for admission to the project must be the existence of a schizophrenic illness for a period of five years or longer and a history of failure in all prior treatments."[39] Despite these stiff criteria, 24 out of 35 patients treated over a three-year period remained well at the time of his report a year later.

The more common approach to allergy as a cause of schizophrenia involves determination by the clinical ecologist of the specific allergies affecting the patient, generally using sublingual or individual food testing. The sensitivity may be not just to the foods themselves but to molds commonly found on foods. "Allergic reactions to several molds have been observed to evoke psychotic cerebral allergic reactions in some schizophrenic patients."[40] There are molds common to all the cereal grains so that a reaction to more than one may be to the molds rather than the grain itself.[51] In everyday life though, avoiding the grains also avoids their molds.

Philpott maintains that "some of the most tenacious and severe phobias, obsessions, compulsions, delusions, and perceptual distortions do occur due to allergic and toxic reactions of the central nervous system."[42] He has found, however, that even though a psychiatric condition may be based on allergy, the patient may need counseling or re-education to overcome inappropriate responses learned during the period of illness. Orthomolecular psychiatrists will also use vitamin therapy, and, if needed, some of the medications and treatments of more conventional psychiatry. Interestingly enough, one of the vitamins used in large doses from the beginning of what was then called megavitamin therapy is niacin. A recent article mentions that this vitamin also seems to have an effect on allergies.[43]

For a family with a severely disturbed member, deliberate food testing can hardly be a do-it-yourself project. It might be workable for a person who is somewhat controllable. A major problem is that so few psychiatrists and mental hospitals use or even are familiar with the possibilities of allergy detection as a means for dealing with disturbed behavior. The number is increasing, however, and a family wishing to locate a doctor or hospital that uses a clinical ecology approach would be advised to contact the Huxley Institute for Biosocial Research in New York City to learn what the nearest possibilities would be. The address is: 1114 First Avenue, New York, N.Y. 10021. The Institute is an informational and not a treatment center. It periodically sponsors national and regional conferences which are open to medical laymen as well as to doctors, and to others in the health professions.

Infantile Autism

Mental illness does not always just strike adults; children can be victims also. There are a number of differences between children who are mentally ill and those who are mentally retarded, neurotic, or hyperactive. Unlike the others, the mentally ill child is largely out of contact with reality. It is like he is locked into a mental world of his own so that he does not really relate to other people. His behavior will be irrational and nonresponsive. Such children are described as being autistic and the condition is referred to as autism.

Treatment of such children has always been very difficult using conventional means because there are so few ways of getting through to or relating to them. Psychologist Bernard Rimland has gathered data indicating that large amounts of some vitamins (C and several of the B vitamins) were helpful for the majority of cases he studied. Of 191 mentally ill children who had been given megavitamin dosages under medical supervision, almost half were "definitely helped," while another 21.5% showed "some improvement." These two categories thus included two-thirds of all the children so treated. This compares with a figure of less than one-third for children treated with conventional drugs.[44]

Dr. Rimland believes that "children loosely called 'autistic' or 'schizophrenic' actually represent a dozen or more different diseases or disorders,"[45] and that further work is needed to separate out and classify these various disorders. A recent paper by Dr. Rimland, Dr. Philpott, and Donna Calvera, the mother of an autistic child, gives evidence that, when this separating-out process has been

148

done, it will likely turn out that a cause of at least some infantile autism is allergy.

Angela Calvera, the little girl reported on, appeared to be completely normal physically. However, as described by her mother she was "locked in a world unknown; unreachable."[46] At age three she was "totally nonverbal." She could not tell her parents "her needs, where she hurt, or anything." Her parents were forced to withdraw her from a college day care center. "Angela also became afraid of things. A crack in a wall or a corner in a ceiling would terrify her. She would run out of the room in hysterics, just to abruptly turn and stare wide eyed and shaking at the spot on the wall that had frightened her so."[47] She did relate to a younger brother to some extent but hardly at all to adults. Learning of Dr. Philpott, the family had Angela undergo a five-week period of diagnosis and treatment for allergy at his clinic. The basic method used was the individual food feeding test after four days avoidance of the food as described in the previous chapter, but supplemented with frequent monitoring of Angela's blood sugar levels, urine and pulse rate.

She turned out to have a number of severe allergies. "She would be peaceful before eating wheat, for instance, but within fifteen minutes after ingesting it, the color drained from her face, she broke out in a sweat, and with eyes half closed, she went into a stupor."[48] She had a similar reaction to oats, which necessitated her sleeping it off for the afternoon. Several kinds of fruit sent her blood sugar levels far higher than the normal top of 160 after eating; apricots and apples producing an almost incredible reading of 400. She also was sensitive to some food colorings and chemicals. Eliminating the guilty foods from her diet and having her eat the safe foods on a rotating basis, so that no one food was eaten often enough to produce further sensitivities, plus supplementing her diet with substantial amounts of vitamins quickly led to a profound change in her behavior.

Even though she was going on four years of age, it had not been possible to toilet train her, but she made considerable progress even during the five-week testing period. Soon after that she was fully trained. "Each day has brought new subtle changes in Angela. It's as if she is slowly waking from a deep sleep. For the first time she is taking interest in what people are doing around her." She started playing with toys appropriately and seeking out the companionship of others. Her mother wrote: "For the first time we really feel like a family and it's wonderful."[49] She started learning to communicate with others, first with sign language and then verbally. Despite attention from specialists at UCLA, she had made no progress until treatment by Dr. Philpott for allergy.

Dr. Philpott makes it clear that Angela has not been "cured" of her condition but, rather, that it has been learned what substances she must avoid and what nutritional supplements she needs to take in order to prevent a recurrence of her symptoms. "She will have to live a carefully regulated life of food rotation, avoidance of certain chemicals, and supernutrition supplements the entire span of her life. Successful living for her will always be a precarious metabolic balance."[50] He hopes that future research will make it possible for her to lead a less regimented life. While such a life will have its hardships, it certainly is far preferable to being the "complete incoherent, hyperactive mess" she was before it was discovered how important allergy was as a cause of her problem and corrective action was taken.

Because this approach has been so little explored, there can be no accurate statistics on the extent to which infantile autism is caused by allergy, but the existence of this one case means there likely are others. This interpretation is strengthened by the finding of the contribution of allergy to adult mental illness, which can not be completely different from that of children.

Alcoholism

While there are approximately 90 million people in the United States who drink alcohol at least occasionally, for some 90% of these alcohol causes no particular problems. The remainder, however, find that they lose control of their drinking to the point that their lives are affected adversely. There is no simple definition of alcoholism. While psychological compulsion is frequently mentioned as indicating alcoholism, some people may drink compulsively at times but in amounts and in circumstances that do not create either social or medical problems for them. Alcoholism involves, then, compulsion to drink plus the drinking of a large enough amount frequently enough so that the drinking causes problems for the individual and others. Lost jobs, broken homes, financial crises and social stigma are some of the results of alcoholism.

There certainly seems to be not just one physical cause of alcoholism, but rather several causes or conditions that can lead to it. Biochemist Roger J. Williams has shown that alcohol consumption can even be studied in the laboratory with animals. He has done experiments where rats are able to take their choice of either plain water or water containing alcohol. "It has been observed in many laboratories, including ours, that rats on high-quality diets voluntarily consume far less alcohol (also less sugar) than those on deficient diets. In individual rats it has been possible to shift their alcohol consumption up and down at will by deliberately making them deficient in specific vitamins, and then supplying the missing nutrients."[51]

Several doctors have reported quite successful results

151

from using high-protein, low-carbohydrate diets plus substantial vitamin supplementation.[52] Dr. Russel F. Smith in the Detroit area has investigated the effect of niacin on over 500 alcoholics during a five-year period and concluded that the vitamin could benefit about 30% of the total alcoholic population.

How does all of this relate to allergy? I would not try to maintain that allergy can explain all alcoholism. Even for the approaches mentioned here, though, the allergy-addiction phenomenon may be relevant. Most alcohol is made from grain and we have seen that grains are among the most common allergens. A high-protein, low-carbohydrate diet minimizes the consumption of grains and thus interferes with the allergy-addiction state that leads to a continued desire for them, even in the form of alcohol. Niacin, we noted earlier, has an effect upon histamine and has also been used successfully by clinical ecologists in treating schizophrenia.

There is more specific evidence, however. Coca reports a case of an alcoholic man who lost his craving for alcohol when living in a house in Florida which was "scantily furnished and well ventilated." Neither did he have a compulsion to drink when living with his daughter, who was allergic to house dust and had had her home treated to minimize house dust. The man himself was never tested for house dust allergy, but, after having his regular home similarly treated for house dust, found not only that he had no compulsion to drink but also that he could engage in normal social drinking without difficulty. The only time in three years when he felt a need to drink secretly was on a day he had been working with an old dusty mattress.[54]

Randolph did the pioneering investigation on the role of allergy in alcoholism and has since had his work confirmed by other clinical ecologists. They have concluded that alcoholism can be sustained both by an allergic addiction to foods from which alcohol is made or, probably less commonly, by the relief which alcohol can give to general stress caused by allergic reactions to other foods.

The difficulties for an alcoholic sensitive to cereal grains should be evident. Beer and the common types of liquor are all made from one or more of the cereal grains—wheat, rye, barley and corn. Randolph points out that the label may not be very helpful in trying to determine the specific grains that have been used; "straight" rye whiskey, for example, needs to contain only 51% rye, the balance being made up of other grains.[55] Rum is made from sugar cane, another member of the cereal grass family. American and Puerto Rican rum may even contain wine which could affect those sensitive to grapes. An alcoholic who ceases drinking but continues to use foods from which the alcohol is made and for which he has an allergy addiction, can have his desire to drink continually stimulated by those foods. Randolph has found that a very high proportion of his patients who were sensitive to cereal grains got allergic reactions to alcoholic beverages made from those grains. He concluded that this was because grain in the form of alcohol is absorbed by the body so quickly and completely. From all of this it becomes quite clear that the person with allergies should be very cautious about alcohol and that anyone with an alcohol problem should investigate allergy as a causative factor.

References

1. Lear, Leonard, "Exorcising the Demons," *Prevention*, July 1977, pp. 158-9.

2. Feingold, Ben F., M.D., *Why Your Child Is Hyperactive*, Random House, New York, 1975, p. 57.

3. Divoky, Diane, "Toward a Nation of Sedated Children," *Learning*, March 1973, pp. 6-13.

4. Feingold, op. cit., p. 62-3.

5. ibid. p. 62.

6. Divoky, op. cit.

7. Feingold, op. cit., p. 51.

8. ibid. p. 169-70.

9. ibid. p. 9.

10. Lear, op cit., p. 159.

11. Feingold, op. cit., p. 12.

12. ibid. p. 123.

13. ibid. p. 59.

14. ibid. p. 71.

15. ibid. p. 72.

16. Sabo, Ruth, Ph.D., "The 'Feingold Families' are on the March," *Prevention*, Sept. 1976, pp. 172-76; and "Trading in Additives for Tranquility," *Prevention*, Oct., 1977, pp. 122-4.

17. Sabo, op. cit., *Prevention*, Sept. 1976, p. 174.

18. Feingold, op. cit., p. 171.

19. Franklin, Betty, "The Feingold Diet Works Wonders for Problem Kids—Even Pets: An Exclusive Interview with the Allergist Who Started it All," *Let's Live*, August, 1977, p. 120.

20. Kinderlehrer, Jane, "Students do Better with A-Plus Food," *Prevention*, June 1976, pp. 70-73.

21. Mandell, Marshall, M.D., personal communication.

22. Moyer, K.E., Ph.D., "The Physiology of Violence: Allergy and Aggression," *Psychology Today*, July 1975, pp. 76-79.

23. Challem, Jack Joseph, "An Exclusive Interview with 'The Children's Doctor,' Lendon H. Smith, M.D.," *Bestways*, August 1977, p. 18.

24. Reported in the Newsletter of Ohio Chapter of Huxley Institute for Biosocial Research, March 1977; a similar approach is used by Dr. Abram Hoffer, see Scheer, James F., "Kicking the Junk Food Habit: Dr. Abram Hoffer's System," *Let's Live*, August 1977, p. 109.

25. *Huxley Newsletter* cited above.

26. Crook, William G., M.D., *Your Child and Allergy*, Professional Books, Jackson, Tennessee, pp. 6-7.

27. Smith, Lendon H., M.D., *Improving Your Child's Behavior Chemistry*, Pocket Books, New York, 1976, p. 40.

28. ibid., p. 88.

29. Challem, Jack Joseph, "An Exclusive Interview with Dr. Theron Randolph, M.D.," *Bestways*, June 1977, p. 28.

30. Mackarness, Richard, M.D., *Eating Dangerously*, Harcourt, Brace, Jovanovich, New York, 1976, Chapter 1.

31. Newbold, H.L., M.D., Philpott, William, M.D., and Mandell, Marshall, M.D., "Psychiatric Syndromes Produced by Allergies: Ecological Mental Illness," *Journal of Orthomolecular Psychiatry*, Vol. 2, No. 3, p. 84.

32. ibid. p. 85.

33. Mandell, Marshall, M.D., "The Medical Ecology Center: The Ecologic Hospital", in Dickey, Lawrence D., M.D., ed., *Clinical Ecology*, Charles C. Thomas, Springfield, Illinois, 1976, p. 470.

34. Philpott, William, M.D., *Ecological Medicine Manual*, Oklahoma City, Oklahoma, 1975 (mimeographed), p. 22.

35. ibid. p. 23.

36. Challem, op. cit., p. 28.

37. See Mandell, Marshall, M.D., "Cerebral Reactions in Allergic Patients: Illustrative Case Histories and Comments," in Williams, Roger J., Ph.D., and Kalita, Dwight, Ph.D., eds., *A Physician's Handbook on Orthomolecular Medicine*, Pergamon Press, New York, 1977, pp. 130-9.

38. Cott, Allan, M.D., "Controlled Fasting Treatment for Schizophrenia," *Journal of Orthomolecular Psychiatry*, Vol. 3, No. 4, pp. 301-11.

39. ibid. p. 309.

40. Philpott, William H., M.D., "Ecologic, Orthomolecular, and Behavioral Contributions to Psychiatry," *Journal of Orthomolecular Psychiatry*, Vol. 3, No. 4, p. 358.

41. Philpott, *Ecological Medicine Manual*, p. 9.

42. Philpott, "Ecologic, Orthomolecular, and Behavioral Contributions to Psychiatry," op. cit., p. 360.

43. Newbold, Philpott, and Mandell, op. cit., p. 91.

44. Rimland, Bernard, Ph.D., "An Orthomolecular Study of Psychotic Children," *Journal of Orthomolecular Psychiatry*, Vol. 3, No. 4, p. 375.

45. ibid. p. 374.

46. Calvera, Donna M., Rimland, Bernard, Ph.D., and Philpott, William H., M.D., *Angela Is Coming Home: Case History of Ecologic Diagnosis and Treatment of an Autistic Child*, Oklahoma City, Oklahoma, October 1976, mimeographed, p. 1.

47. ibid. p. 2.

48. ibid. p. 6.

49. ibid. pp. 6-7.

50. ibid. p. 11.

51. Williams, Roger J., Ph.D., *Nutrition in a Nutshell*, Dolphin Books, New York, 1962, p. 85.

52. see Adams, Ruth and Murray, Frank, *Body, Mind and the B Vitamins*, Larchmont, New York, 1972, Chapter 6; Cheraskin, E., M.D., D.M.D., and Ringsdorf, W.M., Jr., D.M.D., M.S., *New Hope for Incurable Diseases*, Arco Publishing Co., New York, 1971, Chapter 5; Clark, Michael, "The 'Cocktail' that Gets Them Off the Bottle," *Prevention*, Feb. 1976, pp. 126-33.

53. Smith, Russell, F., M.D., "A Five-Year Field Trial of Massive Nicotinic Acid Therapy of Alcoholics in Michigan," *Journal of Orthomolecular Psychiatry*, Vol. 3, No. 4, pp. 327-31.

54. Coca, Arthur F., M.D., *The Pulse Test*, ARC

Books, New York, 1959, pp. 125-6.

55. Randolph, Theron G., M.D., "The Role of Specific Alcoholic Beverages," in Dickey, op. cit., pp. 321-33.

CHAPTER 7

Our Chemicalized Environment

ALTHOUGH OUR PRIMARY interest is food allergy, we shall need to deviate somewhat in this chapter and take a brief look at ways in which people can be affected by other materials in their environment. Some of these overlap with our food supply, as food additives and residues of insecticides or herbicides (weed killers). Other substances operate independently of food. Again, as in so many aspects of allergy covered here, we are indebted to that great research trailblazer, Dr. Theron Randolph, whose 1962 book, *Human Ecology and Susceptibility to the Chemical Environment,* presented a comprehensive treatment of the subject. Interest in the environment only became popular around 1970, but since then many people, both professional and lay, have become seriously concerned with environmental issues.

There are some 30,000 chemicals in use today,[1] with thousands in our food supply. "To illustrate how far out of hand things are, the government does not even know how many additives are being used or by whom, or for what; official estimates range from three thousand to ten thousand."[2] Between 1958 and 1974 government approval was granted to over 3,000 additives and nearly 1,000 were put on the GRAS (generally recognized as safe) list. Governmental acceptance gives no assurance, however, that future evidence will not show that an approved substance actually is harmful in one way or another. There are quite a number of additives which were thought to be safe at one time that are no longer permitted.

Many questions related to health are concerned with these chemicals—the extent to which they may be cancer-causing, whether they can do harm genetically, the effects they may have on species of plants and animals that we depend upon, how they may interact with each other both in our bodies and as environmental pollutants, etc. These are serious matters in their own right but not within the scope of this book.

In the way in which they affect humans, chemicals may be classified as allergens, irritants or toxins (harmful or poisonous substances). Allergens are substances which are normally harmless but which affect some people adversely because of idiosyncrasies of those individuals. Substances which are toxins or irritants, though, have been thought of as affecting all people pretty much the same way, their effects coming from the way they influence life processes. This distinction is becoming clouded, however, as a result of investigation of responses to a number of chemicals in the food supply. While most pesticides and herbicides are clearly recognized as toxins, government policy is to permit small amounts as residues on foods on the assumption that these will not be harmful. But beginning with Dr. Randolph, clinical ecologists have found that some people do get allergic reactions to trace amounts of chemicals in or on foods.

Dr. Mandell informed me that he is currently doing research on responses to such chemicals as DDT, dieldrin, and 2-4-D and has studied 60 patients so far. He has found that some individuals have a reaction to an amount of these chemicals equaling as little as one millionth of the quantity considered by the federal government to be a tolerable amount to consume as residues on food during a normal meal. Of course there is the question of whether the permitted amount is actually safe on a long-range basis, but that is another issue. Here we are noting the fact that some individuals have serious allergic reactions to food chemical residues that are tolerated by the majority of people.

Chemical allergens can produce practically any symptom that food allergens can. Some of the symptoms exhibited by cases mentioned in Randolph's book are: coughing, asthma, rhinitis, bronchitis, canker sores, hives, fever, abnormal weight gains, loss of appetite, headaches, muscle cramps, arthritis, bursitis, aching and stiffness of muscles and joints, and such psychological-behavioral symptoms as chronic fatigue, irritability, poor concentration, dizziness, mental confusion, tenseness, nervousness and fainting.

In a case reported on by Dr. Mandell, a 10-year-old girl staggered out of the girl's lavatory at her school so confused and disorganized that she walked into the wall and did not recognize her teacher or even her mother who was called to come. Some teachers thought she had taken a drug in the lavatory. Eventually it was found that she was extremely allergic to the pine oil which had been used in the cleaning solution in the lavatory.[3]

She was also sensitive to the fluid used in the school duplicating machine and to the solvent in felt-tipped marking pens, getting nauseous and being unable to concentrate. Imagine her feelings when given a freshly run-off assignment and told to work hard at it!

If the list of possible symptoms is long, a compilation of possible chemical allergens would be myriad. It would include all the various chemicals which find their way into our food supply in the forms of insecticides, perservatives, flavor enhancers, substances to retain moisture in foods or to keep them from absorbing moisture, bleaching agents, emulsifiers and thickeners, materials to increase or decrease foaming in liquids, and to alter the texture of solids, curing agents, as well as the colorings and flavorings which Dr. Feingold has emphasized. Some materials, usually preservatives, are added not to the foods but to the packaging and are absorbed from that by the food. Food can also absorb from plastic wrapping or waxed paper and from the lining of metal cans.

Between 1955 and 1975 the amount of additives in our food supply more than doubled to reach an average of five pounds per person.[4] A tiny fraction of a gram may be all that is required to affect a person sensitive to a substance. Chemicals in foods can complicate the problem of trying to determine food allergies. Randolph found that frequently patients were sensitive not to the food itself but to chemicals it contained. This would be most likely with fruits treated with insecticides. Where a patient could eat an organic, unsprayed apple without consequence he might be made ill by an ordinary commercial apple.

An article by Beatrice Trum Hunter provides an example of the problem of additives in foods showing how another chemical has recently been added to a basic food which is ordinarily considered as unprocessed.[5] The substance is papain, which is used as a meat tenderizer with beef, but sometimes also with ham and poultry. Papain meat tenderizer has been available for years for home use, usually combined with other seasonings. Now, however, the government permits it to be added to meat prior to sale, the commercial advantages being obvious; many more cuts of meat can be sold for grilling.

The tenderizer may be injected into the animal just after slaughter or even before. While the carcass is stamped "tenderized" this ordinarily will not be evident to the person picking out a package of meat at the supermarket. Or prior to packaging the cut of meat may be dipped into a tenderizing solution which is likely to contain MSG also. The trouble, of course, is that both papain and MSG can cause severe allergic reactions for some people. If meat tenderizer is added at home to a cut which has already been treated, the person gets a double dose. Papain may also be used in beer, chewing gum, medicines, tooth powder, face creams and lotions. Papain dust may also be an airborne allergen. While any one use might be tolerated, multiple exposures from a variety of products could decrease a person's tolerance to the point of symptoms developing. In testing for allergy to meat if one got a reaction to supermarket beef, another check could be made with organic beef to make sure the sensitivity was to the meat and not to a papain tenderizer additive.

A vast number of chemicals are airborne and reach us whether we are in the city or out in the country. People who move away from the city in an attempt to escape the polluted air from traffic and industry, find there is a whole other group of chemicals used in rural areas—insecticides, fertilizers, and weed-controlling materials (used along roadsides as well as in agriculture). Diffused widely, sometimes with airplanes, they can practically incapacitate affected individuals. Many chemicals these days are found inside the home and would be the same whether it is on the farm or in the city. Wind can carry urban industrial pollutants so that they can affect sensitive people 75 miles away from the source of the pollution.[6]

From the professional standpoint, Dr. Randolph has had the good fortune to have his practice located in Chicago, where the air pollution is so great that he has been able to learn much from it. One of his patients, who lived in a west side suburb and suffered from several symptoms as a result of air pollution, kept a log of his symptoms and correlated them with weather conditions. When at home he literally could tell which way the wind was blowing from his symptoms, which were minimal only when the wind was from a northerly or westerly direction. Winds from the south or east brought with them the city's industrial pollution and would produce headache, coughing, mental confusion, rhinitis and depression. Even the speed of the wind was relevant. The worst was a slow drifting wind; a rate of over 15 miles per hour would keep the pollutants diluted enough so they did not affect him as much.

Modern developments can result in chemicals being introduced right into the structure of the home itself. One material which has been found to cause trouble for sensitive individuals is plastic foam insulation. When a Hartford, Connecticut newspaper ran an article telling of how one family had developed symptoms after having had plastic foam insulation installed in their home, 20 more families notified the paper that they had also suffered adverse effects from foam insulation.[7] Cellulose insulation, which is made of finely shredded paper, could affect people sensitive either to the paper or the chemicals used to make it fire resistant. Particle board and plywood, which usually both contain formaldehyde, are frequently used in making mobile homes, as are artificial wood decorative parts made of plastic.[8]

One vast family of allergenic pollutants is referred to by the general term of hydrocarbons. It takes in the products of coal and petroleum and includes solids, liquids and gases. Gasoline, diesel and oil are some of the more common hydrocarbon liquids but industry uses a huge number of related "petrochemicals." Solids include a whole array of plastics (Randolph had a patient who was allergic to her colored plastic telephone) and synthetic fabrics as well as roof tar and asphalt used for roads. Also wax coatings used to preserve fruits and vegetables. Hydrocarbon gases include natural and bottled gas and the products of their combustion, as well as the fumes from any of the hydrocarbon solids or liquids. Odors from cleaning compounds, polishes, paints, insecticides would all be included, as would even the tiny amounts of oil evaporating from electric motors in household equipment. Exhaust from autos and buses affects a number of people.

The above refers to items that would likely be found around any average home or neighborhood. When we move into the workplace, the possibilities are simply immense. While factories offer the greatest chances for chemical allergens, even stores and offices can have their share. Chemicals used in copying and duplicating machines, inks, art and decorating supplies, specially treated papers and adhesives can all affect sensitive people. Whether at home or workplace, a chemical allergen may work either through being inhaled or from being contacted by the skin. There are cases where a sensitive person in the family has been affected at home by traces of a substance which were brought home from work on the clothing of another family member.

Not all allergens are synthetic chemicals. Everyday natural substances can produce symptoms too. One man who had allergic rhinitis symptoms at work in an accounting office finally traced his symptoms to fumes from wood shavings in a pencil sharpener that happened to be near his desk. A cooperative office manager arranged for employees to use mechanical pencils and the symptoms ceased.[9] Pine wood, so pleasantly aromatic to many people, and turpentine, which is made from pine trees, can affect people sensitive to hydrocarbons. The probable reason for this is that coal, oil and gas all developed out of ancient trees like the pine.[10]

Cosmetics and medications can contain allergenic

chemicals. Sticks for chapped lips are likely to have a petroleum hydrocarbon base,[11] as well as hair preparations. Synthetic fabrics themselves or natural or synthetic fabrics which have been chemically treated for mothproofing, or to produce a certain finish or for no-ironing qualities, all are potential troublemakers for sensitive people. Some people are even allergic to ordinary newspapers, so that stacks of newsprint around can give them symptoms. In one case described by Dr. Newbold, a young woman consulted him regarding allergy symptoms which developed shortly after she started living with her boyfriend. He was an avid reader and kept stacks of newspapers around in their apartment and the symptoms were eventually traced to these.[12]

Chemical allergens can work addictively the same way as food allergens do.[13] Thus, a person sensitive to a certain allergen and exposed to it regularly may need this exposure in order to feel "normal." If materials are similar chemically or functionally one may substitute for another in maintaining the addiction. Petrochemical hydrocarbons, turpentine, and petroleum-derived alcohol is one such group of similar materials. Mackarness cites the case of a painter who, contrary to his usual custom, took a week vacation from his work and went to the seaside. After two days he started feeling tense and uncomfortable. "Walking along the shore one morning, waiting for the pubs to open, he saw a painter working on the ironwork of the pier and immediately struck up a conversation with him, gratefully inhaling huge lungfuls of air heavy with paint fumes."[14] He quickly felt better and spent considerable time during his vacation talking with the painter and getting his fix on the hydrocarbon fumes. Note that the alternative to smelling the paint was drinking in the pub.

A man known to me is now a recovered alcoholic. His work has been in the building construction area both as worker and contractor. He worked for awhile in northern Michigan where he encountered more pine than in other parts of the country. While working there, which was before he got his alcoholism under control, he found that he drank more heavily than in other places and attributes this to the effect of the pine wood.

One major avenue for the entrance of hydrocarbon fumes into the home comes from the need for heating. Each fuel except electricity offers possibilities for contamination. Fumes from a gas furnace and even from tiny undectable seepage from joints in gas piping can cause a reaction in a sensitive person.[15] Fumes from oil heating equipment and storage tanks will cause problems. Coal also gives off vapors and may additionally be treated with kerosene to minimize dust. Combustion products from coal, oil or gas may escape into the house and produce symptoms. A gas cooking stove is right in the living quarters itself. Regarding it, Philpott says: "Likely the most dangerous instrument in the home is the gas kitchen stove. Many people are chronically sick, either mentally or physically, due to exposure to fumes" from it.[16] Randolph similarly cautions about unvented gas-burning room heaters which are commonly used in the Southwest.[17]

Randolph has found that some people are so sensitive to natural gas that even replacing a gas kitchen range with an electric one in itself was not sufficient. Enough gas would leak from valves and joints in pipes to maintain symptoms. Only removing the gas piping from the house would alleviate the symptoms. Heating for these sensitive people would need to be either electric or a hot water system with the furnace in a room whose air is completely isolated from the rest of the house. Even by the time of Randolp's book in 1962, he had had over 500 patients change their gas ranges for electric ones, the improvement in their condition being well worth the expense involved. Such people also would not want to keep their car in a garage attached to the house because of the air contamination from oil, gasoline and exhaust fumes.

Ironically a patient sensitive to both house dust and hydrocarbons may create one problem in the process of solving another. Plastic mattress covers or rubber or plastic foam mattresses and dacron pillows may be used to minimize house dust exposure. All these, however, have possibilities for causing chemical reactions. Randolph prefers feather pillows laundered several times a year over synthetic pillows such as dacron or foam rubber. Plastic foam or sponge rubber in furniture could also cause symptoms, as could plastic or synthetic upholstery material. The general rule for a plastic is that the stronger its odor, the more likely it is to cause trouble. Warm-air furnace filters may have been treated with a hydrocarbon product to make them capture dust better. Some people would be better off with less hydrocarbon and more dust. Re-usable plastic foam filters may also cause problems.

Sensitivity to "house dust" is not literally to dust, i.e., tiny particles of earth. Rather, it now seems that most of the allergenic qualities of house dust are due to insects or fragments of their dead bodies, a particularly important one being the microscopic-sized house mite. The latter is practically a universal companion of man and is found even in the most fastidious homes, a thought one might not like to dwell upon. Bedding is its favorite habitat. A new cotton-padded mattress or a feather pillow will only cause a reaction in the relatively few people who are specifically sensitive to cotton or feathers. After these have been used for awhile, however, they accumulate house mites and become allergenic to the much higher proportion of people who are sensitive to the insect. These people form the bulk of those allergic to house dust.

There is a product called Dust-Seal made by L.S. Green

Associates, 162 West 56th Street, New York City, 10019 which may be used to control house dust. Dust-Seal is added to water and applied to bedding, upholstered furniture, draperies, etc.—anything that is not laundered frequently. Even dogs and cats may be treated. Except for animals the treatment will last for several years. In my case, over a period of several days I treated carpeting, furniture, and bedding in our home, checking my pulse when I awoke in the morning. I finally completed the job by treating the dining room carpeting one day. The next morning I found that my pulse was 63, whereas before that it had consistently been in the low 70's, and it has remained in the low 60's since then. While my pulse rate was not helpful in detecting food allergies it did respond to airborne allergens.

Nevertheless, Dust-Seal has an oil base and should be approached with caution. Coca recommended it and wrote that he had encountered only one case where a person was sensitive to the product itself. Increased exposure to chemicals generally in recent years could result in more widespread susceptibility than earlier. Before treating the whole house with Dust-Seal, a person should be sure he or she can tolerate it. One way to check would be to treat a piece of cloth with the Dust-Seal mixture and after it has dried hold the cloth over one's nose and breathe through it for awhile to see if there is any sensitivity to the substance. If there is not, it could be helpful to the person sensitive to house dust.

This brief resume does not begin to exhaust either the number of allergens or the ways in which people can come to be affected by them. It is only intended to suggest some possibilities which may be considered as examples by individuals trying to understand their own particular situations. Unfortunately, clinical ecologists have found that food sensitivity tends to go along with sensitivities both to natural airborne allergens such as pollen and house dust and to chemical allergens.[18]

If a fast or uncommon foods test as described earlier does not bring about a reduction in symptoms, there are some things a person can do check for the possibility of sensitivity to chemicals. Even during an uncommon foods test, chemical insecticide or preservative residues on foods could result in continued symptoms, not from the food itself but from the chemicals. Only chemically uncontaminated food from a reliable source could show whether the sensitivity is to the food or to the chemicals. Questions such as the following can help to locate nonfood allergens:

1. Is there a seasonal difference in your condition? Hay fever is an obvious possibility, but the person having it will undoubtedly know it. Having more symptoms during the winter points to house dust or indoor chemicals.

2. Do you have any feelings or reactions, either favorable or unfavorable, when exposed to hydrocarbon smells such as gasoline, fumes from road paving or roof tarring, exhaust fumes from autos in heavy traffic, paint or varnish, newly drycleaned clothes, etc.? Trouble is suggested by anything other than a completely neutral reaction.

3. If symptoms began at a certain time, were there any changes that took place in your work or mode of life at about that time? A change of jobs or work assignment or location could bring a person into contact with new allergens that could affect him or someone else in the family sensitive to an allergen carried home from work. Changes in the home such as starting to use a new product or getting new furniture or carpeting which could be allergenic are possibilities.

4. Is there a difference when you are away from work for several days? As it might take several days for absence from an allergen to make a difference a weekend at home might not reveal anything. A vacation of a week or more would be

more significant.

5. Does being away from home for several days make any difference? Being away from home ordinarily means also being away from the normal work site so that judgment must be used in deciding which is really the important one. It may be neither the home nor the office but the region of the country. I know a mother of a boy with rather severe allergies. While visiting in Greece the boy thrived and was symptomless, but as soon as the plane landed in New York the symptoms returned, "even before we got inside the terminal."

Comprehensive Environmental
Control: The Ecological Unit

The ideal approach to use in tracking down difficult cases of allergy involves the use of an "ecological unit" supervised by a clinical ecologist.[19] Such a unit, as part of a hospital, offers as complete control as possible over every aspect of the patient's environment. The air is specially filtered with activated charcoal and other filters, and air circulation is kept separate from that of the rest of the building. Heating may be either electrical or by radiators to minimize hydrocarbon fumes. Maintenance procedures avoid the introduction of allergens in the form of cleaning compounds, floor waxes, etc. Mechanical equipment is either kept out or designed so that it does not give off fumes and odors.

Furniture avoids the use of plastics, synthetic fabrics and foam rubber. Sheets are all-cotton, have not been treated to make them wrinkle-resistant, and are washed in soap rather than detergent, and have not been dried in a gas dryer which could leave hydrocarbon traces. Synthetic clothing materials, all of which come from hydrocarbons, are banned in favor of cotton, wool and silk. Even plastic slippers and handbags are excluded, as are both natural and artificial flowers. All cosmetic items such as hair preparations, nail polish, deodorants, mouth washes, etc. are prohibited, as well as the use of tobacco. Fresh newspapers and magazines are kept out also. All of these restrictions are for the benefit not only of the individual patient but also the other patients in the unit. The result is that the patient lives in as nonallergenic an environment as it is possible to have. Any such unit should be set up so that it could handle psychiatric patients who might become seriously disturbed temporarily during either fasting or testing periods.

The ecological unit can be useful in detecting both food and nonfood allergens. At about the time of admittance, the patient is given a saline laxative to speed up the process of eliminating allergenic foods from the system. The patient then fasts for several days, consuming nothing but spring water known to be free from chemicals. After this, any food which is given initially is organic and also known to be free from chemicals. If there is no reaction to this, the same food, obtained through normal commercial channels and containing pesticide residues, etc. may be given later to check susceptibility to chemical contaminants. When the necessary testing has been done in the unit, the patient is released to go back to his normal environment. He will then be encountering airborne allergens in an unmasked state where his response at home, in the neighborhood, and at work can be noted.

Unfortunately there are very few such ecological units in the country. Dr. Randolph supervises one with 20 beds in Chicago, which contains almost half the ecological unit beds in the United States.[20] Every even moderate-sized city could benefit from such a unit and an ecologically oriented allergist who could make effective use of it. One obstacle to their introduction, aside from the shortage of clinical

171

ecologists to develop and use them, is the resistance of traditional doctors making up the staffs of hospitals to approve such units for their hospitals. This would involve taking a new approach to illness and its treatment.[21]

To describe an ecological unit is to indicate just how far the average home or workplace is from being ecologically ideal for the susceptible individual. This may suggest to you ways in which you can alter your living quarters so they will be less allergenic. This could be done on a temporary basis to see if it makes any difference in how you feel; if you notice an improvement then you could make more permanent changes. Most modern carpeting is made from synthetic materials so that if your home or apartment has installed carpeting you might not be able to do much to reduce substantially the amount of hydrocarbon contamination in your unit.

If your floors are terrazzo (ideal), wood, or even vinyl tile (this seems to be satisfactory even if it is a hydrocarbon),[22] then you can probably arrange so that at least part of your living unit is relatively nonallergenic. Furniture covered or upholstered with synthetic materials or containing plastic or rubber foam can be stored in one room where the air circulation is kept from the rest of the dwelling unit. A gas stove or water heater in the unit will be a problem, but you can minimize such hydrocarbon exposure by shutting the stove off (including pilot lights) and using an electrical hot plate or appliances for cooking.

Remove household chemicals—cleaning materials, Lysol, waxes, polishes, etc.—from the unit and use only soap rather than detergent for washing and bathing. Toiletries and cosmetics should also be kept out. See if you notice any improvement after several days of such avoidance. Note that you will not be attaining perfect control because you will not be able to eliminate chemicals in the outside air. Also, if you live in an apartment building contamination from chemicals in other units will find their way into yours to some extent. But if you are not supersensitive, the reduction in airborne allergens may be enough to make a real difference.

After at least four days of such minimal exposure, try re-exposing yourself to possible allergens. If you have a gas cooking stove, try sniffing generously in the kitchen with several burners operating. If you have put synthetic furniture, rubber pillows and the like in a room or closet, go in and sniff there for several minutes or until you notice a reaction. If the air has been kept from circulating into the rest of your dwelling unit and if the doors have been kept closed, the air there should have a relatively strong concentration of fumes. Try sniffing different toiletries or cosmetic items and note the effects.[23]

One can use a standardized procedure in sniff testing for chemicals.[24] Using small glass jars that medicines come in (they may be purchased from a pharmacy), place a small amount of cotton in the bottom of each. Then put five drops of the substance to be tested in a jar, seal it, and let it sit for four days. One could test for chlorine by using ordinary liquid laundry bleach such as Clorox, alcohol by using rubbing alcohol, insecticides, and toiletry or cosmetic items which you ordinarily use. If you can get some phenol and formaldehyde, test for these also. Both are very widely used in a variety of household products including detergents, plastics, toiletries, and wood products.

Using a well-ventilated area otherwise free from odors, hold the jar containing the test substance twelve inches from your nose and open it. Take a sniff, then another one five minutes later, and a third in another five minutes. If you notice a reaction at any time during the test, stop it by covering the jar and leaving the area. You have found out what you wanted to know. Count the pulse before each test and five, ten, twenty, and forty minutes after beginning it, looking for an increase in rate as a result of the test. Only test one substance a day this way. If this home testing is inconclusive or if you have chemical sensitivities and simple avoidance procedures do not help, then you should consult a clinical ecologist.

References

1. Feingold, Ben F., M.D., *Why Your Child Is Hyperactive,* Random House, New York, 1975, p. 161

2. Verrett, Jacqueline and Carper, Jean, *Eating May Be Hazardous to Your Health,* Anchor Press/Doubleday, Garden City, N.Y., 1975, p. 13

3. Bricklin, Mark, "Psychiatry is a Sick Science,", *Prevention,* July 1973, pp. 65-6

4. Verrett and Carper, op. cit., p. 24

5. Hunter, Beatrice Trum, "Papain Meat Tenderizers: Objectionable for all and Hazardous for Some," *Consumers' Research Magazine,* Sept 1977, p. 36

6. Randolph, Theron G., M.D., *Human Ecology And Susceptibility to the Chemical Environment,* Charles C. Thomas, Springfield, Ill., 1962, p. 53

7. see *Prevention,* May 1978, pp. 90-1

8. see "Dear Betty Lee," *Let's Live,* June 1978, p. 52

9. Rudolph, Jack A., M.D. and Rudolph, Burton M., M.D., *Allergies: What They Are and What to Do About Them,* Pyramid, New York, 1973, pp. 82-5

10. Randolph, Theron G., M.D., "Domiciliary Chemical Air Pollution in the Etiology of Ecological Mental Illness," in Williams, Roger J., Ph.D. and Kalita, Dwight K., Ph.D., *A Physician's Handbook on Orthomolecular Medicine,* Pergamon Press, New York, 1977, p. 169

11. Philpott, William H., M.D., *Ecologic Medicine Manual,* Oklahoma City, Oklahoma, mimeographed, p. 13

12. Newbold, H.L., M.D., *Cerebral Allergic Reactions*

to Drinking Water, Canadian Scizophrenia Foundation Annual Meeting, Windsor, Ontario, 1977

13. Randolph, *Human Ecology and Susceptibility to the Chemical Environment*

14. Mackarness, Richard, M.D., *Eating Dangerously,* Harcourt, Brace, Jovanovich, New York, 1976, p. 57

15. Randolph, op cit., p. 38

16. Philpott, op. cit., p. 13

17. Randolph, op. cit., p. 42

18. see, for example, Mackarness, op. cit., p. 106

19. see Dickey, Lawrence D., M.D., ed., *Clinical Ecology,* Charles C. Thomas, Springfield, Ill., 1976, pp. 70-85 and 86-106; also Randolph, Theron G., M.D., "Ecologic Orientation in Medicine: Comprehensive Environmental Control in Diagnosis and Therapy," in Williams and Kalita, op. cit., pp. 121-9.

20. Mandell, Marshall, M.D., "The Medical Ecology Center: The Ecologic Hospital," in Dickey, op. cit., p. 466

21. ibid. p. 467

22. see Randolph in Dickey, op. cit., pp. 70-85

23. see Philpott, op. cit., and Randolph in Williams and Kalita, op. cit., pp. 121-9

24. Ludeman, Kay and Henderson, Louise, *Allergy Handbook*, Human Ecology Research Association, Dallas, Texax, 1978, pp. 15-16

CHAPTER 8

Hypoglycemia, Allergy and the Pancreas

The Traditional View of Hypoglycemia

ONE CONDITION, WHICH was first reported in the medical literature in the 1920s, has largely been ignored by conventional doctors since then, but which has gotten much attention in recent years from orthomolecular doctors and others in the health movement, is functional or reactive hypoglycemia, also called low blood sugar. Althought apparently different from allergy physiologically, it has a number of outward similarities and, as we shall see, some intriguing actual relationships to allergy. So while the discussion of hypoglycemia may seem to be a digression it is very appropriate for our concern with allergy.

In this chapter we will look at the commonly accepted view of functional hypoglycemia as it has become known in the health movement. Then we shall see how clinical ecology is raising new issues and providing new answers concerning hypoglycemia.

Like allergy, hypoglycemia can cause a wide variety of symptoms and mimic a considerable number of other diseases. One book on the subject lists more than 40 conditions or symptoms which were found to be attributable to hypoglycemia. As with allergy, these symptoms covered a wide range of physical and mental-emotional conditions ranging from nervousness, depression, confusion, blurred vision and fainting to indigestion, headaches, muscle and joint pains and obesity. Before their troubles were traced to hypoglycemia, patients had been diagnosed as mentally retarded, neurotic, alcoholic, diabetic, asthmatic, menopausal, etc.[1] The alert reader will have noticed that some of these symptoms are also the same as those which have been traceable to allergy.

Like allergy, hypoglycemia has not generally been recognized by most doctors as a common condition. It is readily detectable by a standard laboratory test, a glucose tolerance test, which is continued for five or six hours. Yet most doctors do not even think to administer a five-hour glucose tolerance test; if they test for blood sugar at all, it generally is a single test in the morning after a 12-hour fast or one which monitors blood sugar level for only two hours, which will detect diabetes.

In order to understand both the test and the condition itself, it is necessary to know just what hypoglycemia is. It might seem that if the person has low blood sugar all that would be needed to improve the condition would be for him or her to eat more sugar. Actually, what is needed is exactly the opposite! Low blood sugar is thought to result from eating too much sugar and other refined carbohydrates such as white flour. These are so quickly absorbed into the system that the blood sugar level quickly skyrockets to abnormally high levels. Glucose is crucial for the functioning of the brain and the body does not take lightly either abnormally high or low levels of glucose in the blood stream. It has means for both raising and lowering abnormal blood sugar levels to keep the level within the proper range.

When food is digested, part of it is broken down into glucose which goes into the blood stream; a reasonable amount of excess glucose can be transformed into glycogen by the liver and stored in that form. Later, when the glucose level goes down the liver converts the glycogen back into glucose and releases it into the blood stream so that the vitally important glucose level can be maintained within the proper range. I referred above to a reasonable amount of excess glucose. How can one get an unreasonable amount and what happens then?

We need to look at one of the three major types of food, the carbohydrates (the other two types being the fats or oils and the proteins). While many doctors and nutritionists do not pay much attention to the implications of the different kinds of carbohydrates, believing that a carbohydrate is a carbohydrate, orthomolecular doctors place much emphasis upon the distinction between the simple and the complex carbohydrates. Remembering that orthomolecular means right molecules, if ever that term is appropriate it is here. The complex carbohydrates are those in long complicated molecules which are only slowly broken down and absorbed by the body during the digestion process. It is not that they are hard to digest, they are long to digest. Consequently, their food value is absorbed slowly and over a prolonged period by the body and so causes no problems for the mechanism that maintains the blood sugar level. Whole grain cereals and most vegetables would be in the complex carbohydrate category.

The simple carbohydrates, on the other hand, are quickly digested and absorbed by the body, almost instantaneously in the case of ordinary sugar. Within a very short time after eating, the body is flooded with sugar and the alarm goes out. This calls into action the means used by the body to deal with excess glucose, the production of insulin by the islands of Langerhans in the pancreas. Indeed, even before we swallow our first mouthful at a meal, the body has anticipated the coming glucose and started to produce insulin.[2] The insulin, in effect, burns up the excess sugar (and results in it being stored as fat) which brings the blood sugar level back to normal, at least if everything is working properly.

The trouble is that this mechanism was never designed to be subjected to the abuse inflicted upon it by our modern highly processed refined foods. Primitive man, even people living in traditional peasant societies, which were almost universally the only ways of life there were until the 19th century, had very little access to simple carbohydrates. Some fruits are high in these, but they would only be available for a brief period during the year, not long enough to cause trouble. Such people could not afford to squander part of their food supply by refining out only part of the food value and wasting the rest. Also, they did not have the technological means to do so.

Many people in our modern industrial society are living on a sugar roller coaster, however. A breakfast of fruit juice, Danish pastries or white toast (probably with jam) or most supermarket cold cereals (even most "natural" cereals) contains a very high proportion of simple carbohydrate. The caffeine in coffee stimulates the liver to release its stored glycogen, thus depleting its reserves and, if it is drunk with sugar, this adds to the amount of simple carbohydrate. The insulin is called out to handle the excess glucose resulting from all these simple carbohydrates but, because of the emergency nature of the reaction, too much insulin may be produced, resulting in a too-low blood sugar level, which makes the person feel hungry by the middle of the morning. Wanting a quick "pick-up" he or she then has more coffee and a sweet pastry which will last until noon, and so it goes for the rest of the day.

They hypoglycemic has been viewed as someone whose pancreas has been undone by all of this so that it has become oversensitive, pouring out too much insulin in response to excess sugar in the blood stream, so that the sugar level of the blood is reduced not just to normal but to such dangerously low levels that there is not enough sugar to fuel the brain properly and dizziness, confusion and even unconsciousness can result. Short of this, irrational and aggressive behavior and/or a variety of physical symptoms may be produced by hypoglycemia.

Alcoholism is another condition that seems to be caused by hypoglycemia in at least some people. Mention was made in an earlier chapter about how high-protein, low-carbohydrate diets were part of a method that has been used successfully in treating alcoholism. In the body, alcohol seems to work in a fashion similar to sugar. Both are absorbed very quickly after being ingested and both can rapidly raise the blood sugar level. As the brain must have enough blood sugar in order to function, it will force even "irrational" behavior upon the person in order to keep the blood sugar level up. As alcohol will meet this need, the compulsive nature of alcoholism is understandable. While one might substitute sweets for the alcohol, these would keep the person on the blood sugar roller coaster that sooner or later would likely lead the person back to alcohol again. What is needed is rather for the person to get a normally stable blood sugar level by avoiding the simple carbohydrates, making sure all vitamin and mineral needs are met, and as we shall see, avoiding allergens.

Detecting and Correcting
Hypoglycemia

Testing for hypoglycemia is not difficult. The patient has his blood sugar level checked and then drinks a standard quantity of a sugary syrup. His blood sugar level is then checked at least once an hour for five or six hours afterward. Practically everyone will show some rise in blood sugar level during the first hour. The average person will soon produce just enough insulin to bring the level back to normal. The diabetic will soar to a high level and remain abnormally high. The hypoglycemic's level will also usually increase at first but, instead of retreating just to normal, it will continue to fall so that after four or five hours it is well below normal and the person is experiencing physical or psychological discomfort. In some cases the reaction is so rapid and severe the test must be terminated during the third or fourth hour by giving the patient fruit juice or some other quickly absorbed simple carbohydrate. (Note: While taking something sweet is not an appropriate treatment for hypoglycemia, it may be necessary in an isolated emergency situation).

In practice, there are several type of blood sugar curves that indicate hypoglycemia, including a pre-diabetic type of curve and a "flat" curve. Just as important as the blood sugar level on an absolute scale is the overall trend for the person and the rate at which the level falls. A sudden decline from a high to an average level may produce the same kinds of symptoms that are produced by a low level on an absolute basis. Conventional doctors who have not had much experience with or interest in hypoglycemia may not be aware of the variety of curves indicating hypoglycemia, and may think that unless the blood sugar level reaches some arbitrary low point, such as 50, the patient does not have low blood sugar.

Treatment, even for the most severe hypoglycemic, is simplicity itself, if making major changes in one's diet may be called simple. All that is required is for the person to avoid sugar, white flour and other simple carbohydrates in the diet. Without these to set off excess insulin production by the pancreas, the blood sugar level quickly normalizes itself and the person's symptoms depart and mental outlook and energy level greatly improve. The hypoglycemic person is also advised to have a low-carbohydrate snack mid-morning, mid-afternoon, and at bedtime—a glass of milk, cheese, a handful of nuts, etc., so that there is a more constant supply of food coming into the system which minimizes fluctuations in the blood sugar level. There are a number of good books on the subject and the reader who wants more detailed information and specific diet recommendations is referred to them.[3]

Despite the prevalence of the condition, the ease of diagnosis, and the sureness of the treatment, functional hypoglycemia has largely been ignored by conventional doctors. One reason that has been suggested is that there is no profitable miracle drug which can be heavily promoted by the pharmaceutical companies so that doctors would be encouraged to look for the disease and treat it. I have heard of cases where even when doctors gave a five-hour glucose tolerance test and diagnosed the patient as having hypoglycemia their only response was to prescribe tranquilizers for the patient!

Sometimes the medical diagnosis and treatment can have legal implications. In one case, which came before the court in the Cleveland, Ohio suburb of Shaker Heights, a man was being denied unemployment insurance by one of the country's large insurance companies, the justification being that there was nothing physically wrong with the person keeping him from working but that he was psychoneurotic. The man had lost his job because of severe dizziness, headaches, indigestion and extreme weakness. One doctor who testified on behalf of the insurance company did not consider a five-hour glucose tolerance test necessary because "Hypoglycemia clinical syndrome is not a serious syndrome. If the individual will eat more than three times a day or take any form of sugar, that will alleviate attacks." He also testified, "Hypoglycemia is relatively mild all the time. It is never very serious unless it is associated with certain organic diseases."[4] The doctor actually recommended that the man smoke a cigarette when an attack came on (because tobacco, like coffee, stimulates the release of stored sugar from the liver).

Dr. John M. Baron of Cleveland, who had examined and successfully treated the man, testified that his troubles were due to hypoglycemia and that the recommendation to meet an attack of the condition by eating sugar would only make it worse later by causing additional insulin to be released. Dr. Baron certainly would not agree with the recommendation that a person smoke more cigarettes as a treatment for a disease! Had the other doctor, Harold Barker, had his way the patient would have embarked on a long, expensive and ultimately fruitless course of psychiatric treatment (which the insurance would not pay for). Actually, the court decided in favor of Dr. Baron and the patient and thus established a legal precedent for the handling of hypoglycemia cases.

A particularly vivid account of one woman's experience with the condition is given in a little book she wrote describing the 12 years during which she was afflicted with blackouts, rapid heartbeat, amnesia, migraine, fatigue, epileptic-like spells, stomach pain, overeating and weight gain. One night after eating heavily of sugar cookies and coffee at a friend's apartment in New York City, she took the subway home: "I hadn't been seated on the train more than a few minutes when torrents of panic engulfed me. I grabbed the undersides of the seat to keep myself from pulling the emergency cord, claustrophobia choking me so I could hardly breathe. Thirty nightmarish minutes later I was up on the street hugging the sides of the buildings, my hand clutching my heart. Inside my apartment I paced the floor for an hour, a terrible sense of impending danger gripping me."[5]

Her difficulty in getting along with people, another result of hypoglycemia for her, and her inability to work regularly led to loss of jobs and other difficulties. Finally, she just happened to hear about hypoglycemia on a radio broadcast one day and quickly went out and got a book on the subject. Adopting the low-carbohydrate antihypoglycemia diet, which was originally developed in 1924 by Dr. Seale Harris and was described in the book, she quickly became normal. "My recovery, after a few weeks on the Seale Harris diet, was truly miraculous. I doubt, if in the annals of medical history, there was ever a malady so severe and of such long duration that was cured so quickly."[6]

This is all very interesting, but how does it relate to allergy? The answer is that despite the apparent physiological differences between low blood sugar and allergy, there are many functional similarities. For one thing, there are a number of reports in which people with allergies no longer were bothered by them after going on an anti-hypoglycemia diet. This could be because they were allergic to the foods which were forbidden in the diet for low blood sugar. On the other hand, the relationships between the two conditions could be more complicated than that.

We have seen how allergy symptoms develop when stage III of the general adaption syndrome is reached, a stage which is associated with the deterioration of the adrenal glands. Yet the high-protein, low-carbohydrate anti-hypoglycemia diet is just the kind "to place the least amount of strain on the adrenals,"[7] which would give them the maximum opportunity to rebuild themselves.

It is curious also to find that a number of books concerned with one of these conditions devote space to a consideration of the other. Thus, Low Blood Sugar and You by Fredericks and Goodman contains two discussions about allergy and its possible relationship to hypoglycemia. An earlier work by Abrahamson and Pezet on low blood sugar also goes into considerable detail concerning the interesting relationship between asthma and diabetes or hyperglycemia. Individuals may either have either diabetes or asthma; the two conditions are hardly ever found in the same person, although one or the other may affect members of the same family, indicating that the two conditions have a similar genetic basis. Asthma, of course, is one of the classic allergy diseases, but an asthmatic who develops diabetes will find that he is "cured" of the asthma, which is associated with low blood sugar.

Similarly, Judge Blaine's book, *Goodbye Allergies,* bases its approach on improving adrenal function with a heavy emphasis on an anti-hypoglycemia diet. In an introduction to this book, Dr. Sam E. Roberts, an emeritus professor at the University of Kansas Medical School, Kansas City, wrote about allergy: "Hypoglycemia (low blood sugar) is nearly always present." Judge Blaine advocates an approach developed by Dr. John W. Tintera which involves shots of adrenal cortical extract (ACE) as well as diet. The ACE is thought to take over the job of the adrenal cortex, allowing it to rest and rebuild so that it can make the person less susceptible to allergens. However, the FDA has recently suspended its approval of ACE, at least temporarily, claiming that newer and less natural preparations are more effective, so that even if one could find a doctor willing to administer the substance, it would be difficult to obtain. Yet, Dr. Mandell told me that many patients of his have found it very helpful. He has gotten the maximum benefit when it has been supplemented with vitamins.

A New View of Hypoglycemia

A whole new area of exploration has been opened up

into the tangled web of cross-relationships between hypoglycemia and allergy by the work of clinical ecologists. Following up on leads supplied by Dr. Mandell, Dr. Philpott has been investigating the effect on blood sugar levels of foods being tested in deliberate feeding tests as described earlier. He has found cases where hypoglycemia has been produced by foods containing little or no carbohydrate, and others have had similar results.

Such findings are truly astounding because, according to the traditional view of hypoglycemia, only the quickly absorbed simple carbohydrates should be capable of causing serious alterations in the blood sugar level. Philpott cites the case of a man allergic to milk whose blood sugar level sank to an extremely low point two hours after eating a test portion of cream cheese, a food which contains only two per cent carbohydrate. In describing these results Philpott wrote: "The assumption that these disordered carbohydrate reactions will be in response to carbohydrate only is not valid. Testing reveals that they occur to any type of food and that the central cause is that of being allergic to or allergic in a specific way to a specific food whether fat, protein or carbohydrate. In this case the hypoglycemic response was to cream cheese which is largely a protein and fat food."[8] This is truly a bombshell in the whole hypoglycemia picture.

Dr. Philpott is not alone in his view about a relationship between allergy and hypoglycemia. Dr. H.L. Newbold of New York City turned from the practice of psychiatry to a general practice emphasizing a nutritional approach as a result of his own personal experience.[9] A hypoglycemic with problems of general ill health, obesity and depression, he analyzed his own condition after conventional medicine proved unable to help him and concluded that he should go on an anti-hypoglycemia diet. Shortly after starting the high-protein, high-fat, low-carbohydrate diet, his troubles cleared up, the evidence being not just in a subjective feeling of health and energy but in objective measures such as the loss of 50 pounds down to a normal weight and a decline in blood cholesterol from 312 to 149.

It is not really surprising to find out that Dr. Newbold also has a number of allergies, including a sensitivity to some types of drinking water. While the anti-hypoglycemia diet has helped his health generally he still needs to avoid a number of food allergens.[10] He treats his patients with individualized programs of testing and treating for allergies, vitamin and mineral supplementation and recommendations concerning diet. Thus he is a doctor who has had personal experience with both hypoglycemia and allergy and who frequently encounters these conditions among his patients. He has stated that he considers allergy to be a more basic condition than hypoglycemia and that he believes that practically all hypoglycemia is the result of allergy.[11]

Dr. Marshall Mandell was one of the earliest investigators of the effect of allergens on blood sugar levels and has come to the conclusion that the classic type of functional or reactive hypoglycemia caused by excessive consumption of simple carbohydrates may not even exist as a disease entity. In a paper which discusses this subject, he recognizes that many people have been helped by the anti-hypoglycemia diet but believes that in such cases it is because the diet eliminated foods which were allergenic for the individual.[12] It is not that the diet protects the pancreas from too much sugar which would cause it to overproduce insulin, but that it eliminates allergic reactions. More recently he said that "people have used hypoglycemia as a handle to describe addictive and allergic reactions."[13]

Mandell observed early in his research that patients' reactions to different foods are specific rather than being a generalized reaction to "starches" and "sugars". He states:

"Every 'hypoglycemic' subject having a 'carbohydrate' intolerance does not have an across-the-board problem with all carbohydrates."[14] He emphasizes that "sugars" are different depending upon what they are made from, and notes, as others have also, that cane and beet sugar can produce different reactions. Glucose, one type of sugar, may be made from potato or from various cereal grasses, frequently corn. When we consider that glucose is the sugar ordinarily used in glucose tolerance tests and that corn is one of the most common allergens, we can see how a reaction to the glucose could be due to sensitivity to the food from which the glucose is made rather than, as has been traditionally believed, simply to the sugar. Even though the chemical structure of two sugars may be the same, "each of the sugars carries species-specific plant material from the source of its origin...."[15] The problem of sugars seems to be more complex than was thought.

Dr. Mandell also cautions about the traditional anti-hypoglycemia diet, even while noting that it undoubtedly has helped many individuals. He is concerned that frequent exposure to the proteins specified in the diet can aggravate a tendency to react to those foods, and can even cause new sensitivities to develop to those frequently-eaten foods. With patients who had been following the anti-hypoglycemia diet but were still having difficulties, provocative food tests used by Dr. Mandell showed repeatedly that the symptoms were due to the protein foods which the subject had been eating every day. As he put it, "many proteins which had been eaten to relieve 'hypoglycemia' were demonstrated to be causing the symptoms they were expected to control.[16]

What does all this mean for the person confronting problems of allergy and hypoglycemia? The conclusion which suggests itself from the evidence we have reviewed here is that allergy is the more fundamental of the two and that one should find out what substances one is allergic to, because even noncarbohydrate foods can produce hypoglycemic reactions. The traditional anti-hypoglycemic diet calls for the regular consumption of such high protein foods as meat and fish, eggs, nuts, milk and cheese, etc. Yet, both eggs and milk are commonly allergenic foods, and others in the diet are not far behind. Before one embarks on a diet heavy with foods allergenic for so many people one should know that these foods can be tolerated. Furthermore, the diet encourages the person to eat a limited number of foods frequently, so that new sensitivities to these foods could develop from overexposure to them.

A newer approach within the conventional perspective of hypoglycemia is a diet which also eliminates the simple carbohydrates but calls for the bulk of the calories to come from the complex carbohydrates—whole grains and vegetables—rather than from protein.[17] These complex carbohydrates are broken down and absorbed slowly by the body just as are proteins. Here again though, caution regarding allergy is in order. Whole wheat can be wonderful for anyone not allergic to it, but wheat is a very common allergen, as are other cereal grains. With this diet as well, sensitivity to foods needs to be kept in mind.

Clinical ecologists recommend against the simple carbohydrates for many reasons, poor nutrition being enough of a reason in itself. When dealing with hypoglycemia, however, they emphasize that first one needs to deal with the problems of allergy. When this is done, the hypoglycemia should be corrected in the process.

A Theory of Allergy

One of the most serious stumbling blocks involving allergy is, as noted in the first chapter, that traditional medicine has lacked an understanding of what causes allergy and has not been able to fit moladaptive reactions to various substances into a neat theoretical scheme except for that of immunology. While such early clinical ecologists as Rinkel and Randolph developed an effective means for detecting allergens (a feeding test after four day's avoidance) and were successful in dealing with their patients' symptoms, they did not have a theoretical explanation for what they were doing or why it worked.

We have already mentioned Philpott's observations on the effects of different kinds of foods upon the blood sugar level of his patients. He has, however, investigated a number of aspects of the body chemistry of patients in situations where he knew just what their status was concerning exposure to allergenic-stressor substances— i.e., after a four-day fast when the person was free of the effects of allergens and at various time periods after exposure to an allergen. Conventional doctors are not in a position to do this because their testing methods are inadequate and they do not take into account that a person can be under the influence of an allergen and yet be symptom-free because of masking. Clinical ecologists are able to see just what the effects on the body chemistry are of exposure to an allergen. Out of this is coming a real understanding of how allergy works.

Dr. Philpott and medical writer Dwight K. Kalita are planning a book which will present research evidence, theoretical explanation and methods of treatment. Their volume should appear sometime subsequent to the publication of this work and so of course is not available for citation here. Dr. Philpott, however, has written a number of papers which he has reproduced and circulated privately and has also given papers at professional meetings. It is from these that I will draw in describing an emerging theory of allergy.

The key body organ involved in allergy is the pancreas,

"which emerges as the initial and most important stress shock organ." The pancreas plays a crucial role in the metabolism of food, producing both enzymes needed for their digesting and bicarbonates needed to provide an alkaline environment for these enzymes to work effectively. The stomach itself produces acid which is necessary for the first stage of digestion of many foods, but then as the food leaves the stomach and enters the small intestine it needs an alkaline medium, which is normally provided by the pancreatic bicarbonate.

Affected individuals, however, will not have a normally functioning pancreas. This may result from an inborn defect (producing a fixed allergy), from various kinds of nonfood stresses such as infection, heat or cold, fatigue or emotion, or from too-frequent contact with foods which stress the pancreas by requiring enzymes it can not readily produce. Thus, at the base of allergy is an inadequately functioning pancreas. The first pancreatic function to be affected in the development of the disease process is production of bicarbonate, second is the production of enzymes, and last and most resistant to interference is the production of insulin, which is another pancreatic function. Bicarbonate inhibition is not across the board, but rather is selective for particular foods. A normal amount of bicarbonate will be produced for nonallergenic foods, while those to which the person is sensitive will inhibit pancreatic functioning.

It has long been known that common adult-onset diabetes, called diabetes mellitus, results from inadequate insulin production so that the body cannot maintain a sufficiently low blood sugar level. The developing theory of allergy maintains that the condition is closely related to diabetes and is an earlier stage of diabetes. As Philpott writes: "The chemistry of [allergy] addiction to foods and the chemistry of the diabetes mellitus disease process are observed to be one and the same." Before a person shows clinical symptoms of diabetes he will have disordered metabolic functioning, which would show up in laboratory tests if appropriate ones were made. This pre-symptom stage is that of *chemical* diabetes mellitus, which is characterized by disturbed acid-alkaline balances in the body and by periods of both hypoglycemia and hyperglycemia (high blood sugar). By the time *clinical* diabetes mellitus develops, most of the insulin-producing capacity of the pancreas has been lost and there is consistent hyperglycemia.

Philpott thus finds himself focusing on the chemical diabetes mellitus process in his attempt to understand allergy. This process in turn can be related to the G.A.S. of Selye described earlier, except that, whereas Selye emphasized the adrenocortical aspects of the G.A.S., Philpott calls attention to the pancreatic "enzyme failure as a point where the stress syndrome begins to fail." The adaptive addiction stage of allergy is that of stage two of the G.A.S. which in turn is the same as the chemical diabetes mellitus stage. To speak of a stage in a process implies that one will go on to another level, but Philpott makes it clear that a person in the chemical diabetes stage may be able to remain there indefinitely without proceeding to actual clinical diabetes so that no inevitable progression is necessary.

If digestion is complete, food is broken down into basic substances usable by the body, amino acids, glucose, etc. However, inadequate pancreatic functioning will result in incomplete digestion so that protein molecules of the food itself which are unusable by the body in that form are absorbed by the intestine and circulate in the bloodstream. There, they can produce an inflammatory reaction in tissue which they contact by causing the body to produce either histamine (which is an immunological reaction) or kinin (which is nonimmunological). Of the two, kinin is more likely to cause pain than histamine because of the effect it has on nerve endings. Based on work both by himself and others, Philpott has concluded that for schizophrenics, two thirds of their allergic reactions are due to kinin rather than histamine.

While the pancreatic enzyme trypsin can stimulate kinin production, other pancreatic enzymes can combat kinin and prevent or reduce inflammatory reactions. Thus, a malfunctioning pancreas can both contribute to inadequate digestion which allows food irritants to enter the bloodstream and to continued inflammation from the resulting kinin through insufficient production of alkaline bicarbonates and of enzymes to control the kinin. An acid condition of the body stimulates the production of kinin, whereas an alkaline condition favors the enzymes which destroy kinin. The level of kinin required to produce an inflammatory reaction varies according to the state of the individual. A person who is poorly nourished, toxic or infected, or who is in the addiction stage, will be affected more by a given level of kinin than he would be otherwise.

Various factors specific to an individual will determine which part or parts of his body will be most affected by allergy-produced inflammation. In the addiction stage, where an allergenic food is eaten regularly the inflammation becomes chronic and injures the tissues. Eventually the adaptation of stage two breaks down and the person enters stage three in which there are observable symptoms of illness. The person goes to a doctor and is diagnosed as having a particular disease, which could be any of the 100-plus conditions mentioned earlier. "The diseases are named according to the tissues involved, the disordered endocrine glands, the autoimmune disorder evoked, or the secondary invading microbes. The diseases produced in this way encompass a long list of common degenerative diseases common to mankind."

Thus, while illness caused by allergy-addiction may be named according to the specific tissue or biochemical process involved, etc., all types trace back to chemical diabetes mellitus in which allergenic foods, chemicals, etc. cause reactions "because they interfere with metabolic processes." Philpott believes that "addictive adaptations to frequently used foods and commonly met chemicals can be as deteriorating to metabolism and tissues as narcotic and alcohol addiction.... It is more correct to talk of an addictive state of metabolism than an addictive substance..." He also considers that "mankind's greatest stressors are addictions to frequently used foods and commonly met chemicals." Allergy, then, is not just a minor little anomaly but rather a disturbance in some of the body's fundamental life processes.

With this as a background we can see what happens during provocative testing after at least four days' avoidance of a substance. During the avoidance period the body reverts to the unadapted first stage in which an allergenic-stressor food or chemical will produce a stronger reaction than during the addictive stage. Reactions during provocative tests are "the diseases in miniature, i.e., acute reactions which are the same as the chronic reactions of the diseases." The acute symptoms of provocative testing are "the building blocks for chronic degenerative disease either mental or physical. Thus acute arthralgia as a test reaction when chronic is named as arthritis...a stuffy nose and/or sinus test reaction when chronic and usually infected is named as chronic rhinitis and/or chronic sinusitis, acute test reactions interfering with or distorting mental functions or emotions are when chronic named as neuroses or psychoses depending on the type of symptoms." The fact that these diseases clear up when the stressor substances are identified and avoided shows their relationship to addiction and the chemical diabetes mellitus stage.

If chemical diabetes mellitus can produce the whole range of allergy-caused diseases, how about clinical diabetes mellitus itself? Traditional medicine views diabetes as due only to disordered carbohydrate metabolism, so that a diabetic taking insulin will adjust his insulin intake to the amount of carbohydrate consumed. In the process of testing patients Philpott has found that for individual diabetics there are some carbohydrates which do not abnormally elevate blood sugar, but that some fats and proteins do, as well as some nonfood substances such as petrochemical fumes and tobacco smoke. His approach is to detect and have the patient avoid all allergenic foods and chemicals, to look for and treat any possible infections, to provide adequate vitamin and other nutrient intake, to control diet to eliminate obesity, and to use pancreatic enzyme and bicarbonate supplementation (which will be described later). These measures frequently make it unnecessary for the diabetic patient to continue taking insulin; those who do need it often can reduce the amount they need to take.

Dr. Philpott's observations have been confirmed in work done by Drs. John E. Potts and Alvin S. Lang of Walla Walla, Washington. Working with seven "poorly controlled obese" diabetics whose condition developed when they were adults, the doctors first had them fast for four days while being monitored. During the fast the blood sugar levels of these diabetic patients decreased to a normal or near-normal level. Provocative testing which followed revealed sensitivities to a number of both carbohydrate and protein foods which elevated the patients' blood sugar levels. When the patients avoided the incriminated foods, their insulin requirements decreased considerably, four of the patients being able to get along without any insulin. The doctors concluded: 'Results suggest that avoidance of incriminated foods may favorably influence the dietary management of diabetes."[18]

Dr. Philpott maintains that as long as the patient is regularly being exposed to allergenic foods and chemicals, it is true that the counts of total calories and carbohydrates in particular can serve as a "rough guide to the insulin need. However as soon as the diabetic is withdrawn from the several selective substances he maladaptively reacts to, then it is no longer true that the insulin needs can be judged by the carbohydrate calories or the total calories." As cautioned earlier in the chapter on testing, diabetics should not experiment with this without medical supervision. Eliminating allergenic foods from the diet and subsequently testing them could sharply alter one's insulin needs.

The biggest problem might come in finding a doctor who would at lease consider it possible that allergy could produce a diabetic state, because traditional medicine does not recognize this possibility. Philpott found that some doctors, even when shown case histories of successfully treated patients or when confronted with their own diabetic patients who no longer had abnormal blood sugar levels, spillage of sugar in the urine, or a need for insulin still denied that allergy could produce a diabetic state. On the other hand, some doctors welcomed the information and considered it worthy of further investigation. In a way, treating diabetes through allergy management is not new. Coca reported successful cases of diabetic treatment in the 1950's,[19] although without the theory and detailed clinical work of the modern clinical ecologists.

References

1. Fredericks, Carlton, Ph.D., and Goodman, Herman, M.D., *Low Blood Sugar and You,* Constellation International, New York, 1969, pp. 20-34.

2. Kipnis, David M., M.D., statement on "Daniel

Foster, M.D.," television program produced by KERA-TV, Dallas, Texas, 1977.

3. Abrahamson, E.M., M.D. and Pezet, A.W., *Body, Mind, and Sugar,* Pyramid Books, New York, 1951; Adams, Ruth and Murray, Frank, *Is Low Blood Sugar Making You a Nutritional Cripple?,* Larchmont Books, New York, 1975; Martin, Clement G., M.D., *Low Blood Sugar: The Hidden Menace of Hypoglycemia,* Arco Publishing Co., New York, 1969.

4. Kalita, Dwight K., Ph.D., "A Legal Triumph for Orthomolecular Medicine," in Williams, Roger J., Ph.D., and Kalita, *A Physician's Handbook on Orthomolecular Medicine,* Pergamon Press, New York, 1977, pp. 223-4.

5. Thienell, G.M., *My Victory Over Low Blood Sugar,* Arco Publishing Co., New York, 1970, p. 14.

6. ibid., p. 85

7. Blaine, Judge Tom R., *Goodbye, Allergies,* Citadel Press, Secaucus, New Jersey, 1965, p. 59

8. Philpott, William H., M.D., "The Significance of Selective Food and Chemical Stressors in Ecological Hypoglycemia and Hyperglycemia as Demonstrated by Induction Testing Techniques," *Journal International Academy of Metabology,* Vol V, No. 1, p. 81

9. Gonzales, Nicholas, "Why This Psychiatrist 'Switched'," *Prevention,* September 1976, pp. 55-60.

10. Newbold, H.L., M.D., stated during his presentation, *Cerebral Allergic Reactions to Drinking Water,* Canadian Schizophrenia Foundation Annual Meeting, Windsor, Ontario, Canada, June 1977.

11. ibid.

12. Mandell, Marshall, M.D., "The Diagnostic Value of Therapeutic Fasting and Food Ingestion Tests In a Controlled Environment," *Journal International Academy Metabology,* March 1975, p. 83.

13. Mandell, Marshall, M.D., personal communication

14. Mandell, "The Diagnostic Value...," p. 84

15. ibid.

16. ibid., p. 86

17. Airola, Paavo, M.D., "Causes of Hypoglycemia," *Let's Live,* May, 1977, p. 81

18. Potts, John E., M.D. and Lang, Melvin S., M.D., *Avoidance Provocative Food Testing in Assessing Diabetes Responsiveness,* paper given at American Diabetes Association Annual Meeting, St. Louis, Missouri, June 1977.

19. Coca, Arthur F., M.D., *The Pulse Test,* ARC Books, New York, 1959, pp. 72-75.

CHAPTER 9

Rotation Diets and Food Family Tables

SOME LUCKY INDIVIDUALS discover that they have a reaction to only a few foods which are easily dropped from the diet. At the other extreme are those with low inherent tolerance who quickly become sensitized to many substances through too-frequent exposure. Yet, the majority of sensitivities are cyclic rather than fixed. This means that most food allergies can be lost through a period of abstinence, as described earlier, and prevented from reappearing by avoiding overexposure through too-frequent consumption of the allergenic foods. One can also prevent new sensitivities from developing by spacing one's exposure to foods that have been tolerated in the past. This can be particularly important when these foods are in a family including other foods to which one has gotten reactions.

The best way to do this is by using a rotation diet. An early form of this, called the rotary diversified diet, was developed by Rinkle back in the 1930's. It could be used for both diagnostic and diet regulation purposes. The basic idea of the modern rotation diet is very simple—to space out the frequency of eating a particular food so that it does not result in the person becoming sensitive to it. Ordinarily, this means eating the food not more than once in every four days. As even this infrequent a rate of consumption may be too much for some foods for some people, a longer interval may be required. Some rotation diets limit foods to once in seven days. Some people may find that a certain food causes trouble if it is eaten oftener than once in a month.

It is possible to acquire new sensitivities on a four-day rotation diet. Knowing that I was sensitive to melons, I was careful about pumpkin and squash, which are also in the gourd family, but did start eating them on my rotation diet, alternating them every other day. The last two times I have had squash, however, I noticed some stomach reactions afterward. This is one of the advantages of the rotation diet—your reactions will be evident and not masked. I shall avoid these vegetables for awhile and then try scheduling them less frequently. The situation for these particular foods is complicated by the fact that canned pumpkin may contain winter squash,[1] so that a person can get more exposure than he thinks. Buckwheat can be a substitute for cereal grasses, but RRZ found that many people became sensitive to it and urged caution in its use.[2]

The ability to lose sensitivity to a cyclic allergen means that you will eventually be able to include foods to which you are now sensitive. A rotation diet will be your best insurance against becoming sensitive to them again, because RRZ found that their patients could rarely go back to an allergenic food to which they had lost sensitivity and eat it oftener than once in three days without becoming resensitized.[3] Remember that the frequency with which a food is eaten is much more important than the amount which is eaten in causing sensitivity, so that substantial quantities of the food every four days are much less likely to cause trouble than small amounts every day.[4] This is fortunate because, as you will see, spacing foods out on a rotating basis limits the number of foods which can be used at any one meal.

If you, like many people, have gotten into a food rut, eating the same few foods over and over again, a rotation diet may be quite unpleasant to contemplate (it was for me), because it calls for a major alteration in your food habits. When you get into it though, you are likely to find that you feel better and that you actually relish the greater variety and possible new foods it calls for.

While I can look back with fond memories to when I felt I could eat anything at any time (and didn't know that this was what was causing my health problems), I accept the fact now that this can never again be, and I cannot now imagine myself eating differently from the way I do. I, who had almost continuous colds before have not had a cold for seven months, and that one came in the middle of the winter after I experimented with eating oatmeal. The previous cold was in the preceding summer just after having returned from three weeks travel in Egypt and Greece, during which time I was not able to follow my diet. Do I find myself agreeing with Coca's view that you don't catch colds, you eat them? Definitely!

Once you understand a few simple principles you will find that it is not hard to make up a rotation diet that meets your particular needs. You could, for example, construct a diet which rotates some foods on a four-day cycle and others on a longer basis.

Given in this chapter are classifications of foods by family for both plant and animal kingdoms. These are presented in two ways, alphabetically by name of the individual food and grouped according to food family. Although I have tried to make the food classification tables quite comprehensive, there still might be some uncommon foods that are not included. For these, a dictionary or encyclopedia might give their biological classification, or your local library could help.

The system used by Dr. Randolph is to permit foods from a particular family to be used on one day, nothing from that family on the next day, then different foods from that family on the following day. For example, one might have peas from the legume family, then no legumes on the next day, and beans on the following day. One could eat more than one food from a particular family at the same meal (thus one might have both peas and navy beans), but then if one had legumes two days later they would need to be different legumes (perhaps soybeans and peanuts). A particular food family is permitted every other day but any specific food is allowed only once every four days. Some foods you may have to limit to once every seven or 14 days, but they can be fitted in with no particular difficulty. You may need to have your basic rotation be on a seven day cycle rather than four days, in which case you would alternate the families on a three- and four-day basis rather than on a two-day basis and space the individual foods seven days apart.

Making Out a
Rotation Diet

The first few times you make out a rotation diet it will seem like a slow, cumbersome process, but as you get used to the procedure and become familiar with food family classifications it will soon become routine. Start by taking a sheet of paper and dividing it into seven columns, one for each day of the week. Then draw two horizontal lines so that the column for each day is divided into three equal parts, one part for each meal for that day. Then start filling in the squares for each meal, consulting the food tables as you go along.

Your selection will depend upon your particular food

preferences and needs to avoid certain foods. A rotation diet is feasible only if you limit the number of foods you have at any one meal, so that fewer different foods but larger quantities of each are the rule. Get used to the idea of only two or three kinds of foods at a time, but having them in larger portions than you may have been used to.

You may have to change some of your ideas about what is appropriate for a particular kind of meal. Dr. Randolph told me that, because of sensitivity to them, he has not eaten cereal grains for 35 years. When I asked him what he had for breakfast he told me that that morning he had oranges and fish. Given that, despite his sensitivities at age 72, he is trim, healthy and alert it is hard to argue with his approach. A food which produces only a minor reaction may be included in the diet. Dr. Randolph mentioned that an hour or so after eating oranges he will sneeze a time or two, but as that seems to be their only effect he still eats them periodically.

Advising on breakfasts is difficult because people vary so greatly in how much, and what kinds of foods they want for that meal. If you can eat fruits you should have little trouble in arranging different ones for the different days. If you prefer cereals and can tolerate them, you will still need to have a non-cereal breakfast every other day because all cereals are in the same family. Buckwheat would be one alternative, being a cereal-like food that is not in the cereal grass family. Also, one could chop up nuts in the blender and eat them like a cold cereal, perhaps with chopped up dried fruit. For some people, both cereals and nuts might have to be excluded. In that case, despite being unconventional, vegetables and meat or fish might be the most appropriate fare for breakfast.

My preference is to schedule the vegetables first and add the meats afterward. With the vegetables, you can arrange a mix of the starchy and non-starchy ones to give an appropriate number of calories. By eating adequate meals at mealtime you should be able to avoid the need to snack between meals, which would complicate the allocation of foods over the cycle.

In making out a sample rotation plan let us start with carrots for Monday evening. These are in the parsley family and if we wanted another starchy vegetable for Wednesday we could schedule parsnips for that day. Celery could also be included in either the Monday or Wednesday meal, along with the carrots or parsnips. Potato could give us a starchy vegetable for Tuesday and sweet potato for Thursday. From the mustard family we could choose broccoli for Monday, cauliflower for Wednesday, Brussels sprouts for Friday, and kale for Sunday. From the legumes we might select beans for Tuesday, peas for Thursday, and lentils for Saturday. We can draw on the composite for a salad every other day, and if these are alternated with legume sprouts (alfalfa, mung beans), one can have raw foods every day. With the addition of fruits, meats and nuts, one can have a well balanced diet, very likely better balanced than a non-rotation diet. The accompanying chart gives a sample rotation diet for a one week period, designed to meet the particular conditions specified. Your diet could be quite different on your particular sensitivities.

A Sample Rotation Diet

Rotation diets will be different for different people because of the foods they may or may not be able to eat, food preferences, regional and seasonal variations, etc. This illustrative diet (Fig. 11) meets the following conditions: No wheat, corn, milk, or milk products. Each permitted fruit, nut, or cereal grain is on a seven-day rotation with at least three-day spacing of their food families. Other foods are on a four-day rotation.

Fig. 11. Sample Rotation Diet

	Breakfast	Lunch	Dinner
Monday	banana, orange, raisins	salmon, salad, with safflower oil dressing* beans, asparagus	broccoli, chicken, carrot, celery
Tuesday	buckwheat cereal, maple syrup		potato, steak, mushrooms
Wednesday	chopped walnut "cereal" with dates	salad, spinach, tuna, sesame oil dressing*	turkey, parsnips, pears
Thursday	grapefruit, oatmeal with cane sugar	peas, squash, mung bean sprouts, peanut oil dressing*	sweet potato, pork chop, tomato
Friday	figs, eggs	large salad with safflower oil dressing*	haddock, Brussels sprouts, carrots
Saturday	chopped almond "cereal," apricots	lentil soup, alfalfa sprouts, soy oil dressing*	potato, lamb, mushrooms
Sunday	plums, millet cereal, cane sugar	beets, chard, sole	chicken, kale, applesauce

* Just the oil base of the dressing is specified. The seasonings added to the oil can be varied according to one's tastes and tolerances.

Following the
Rotation Diet

It takes different enzymes to digest each food, and repeated demands on the body for producing the same enzymes over and over can weaken the enzyme-producing capacity for those enzymes. A rotation diet eases the burden by calling for a variety of enzymes so that none of them have to be produced at too high a rate. The result should be a more adequate supply of enzymes for the foods consumed.

How you prepare each food is, of course, up to you, and altering the means of preparation can in itself introduce variety into the menu. Thus, you might have raw carrot sticks one time and steamed carrots another. Frying introduces another food into the situation, namely the fat or oil in which the frying is done. There would be no problem from this if it is an oil or fat used in the same meal, pork fat from the meat or safflower oil, for example, used also in a salad dressing.

Situations could arise, most likely from eating out or special occasions, that could cause you to deviate from your diet. If you have been following it regularly though, a lapse now and then should not cause any difficulty. Some foods you may feel are safe for you so that you could eat them oftener than every four days. If you are honest with yourself, it could be quite satisfactory to do so. However, it would be a good idea every month or so to go without the food for four days before eating it again just to make sure you have not developed a masked sensitivity to it. Otherwise, eating a food no oftener than once every four days keeps it unmasked, so that if it gives you no reaction you can be sure it is safe for you. By the same token, at least at first, you may stumble upon some additional sensitivities because all the foods you will be eating will have been unmasked. This is why a rotating diet can be both a diagnostic and therapeutic tool.

Any food for which you have a permanent sensitivity should, of course, be excluded from the diet, but not necessarily the whole family from which that food comes. Thus, in the sample rotation diet given here, it is assumed that there is a permanent sensitivity to corn and wheat but that other members of the cereal grass family may be eaten on a rotating basis.

Obviously such a diet rules out much ready-prepared food, which is likely to have too much of a mixture of ingredients. One should be cautious even about simple foods, however. Thus, if one had orange juice one day and pineapple juice another and they were both sweetened with cane sugar, then the system would be broken. With prepared foods one generally does not know whether beet or cane sugar has been used, and there is a strong likelihood of "corn sweeteners." If you find that you fare well on the rotation diet, you may wish to experiment to see if at least some foods can be eaten more often than every fourth day. You will have to judge on the basis of your own experience.

In making out your diet and when preparing and eating foods, do not overlook the food family classifications of incidental foods such as cooking oils, spreads, sauces, dressings and sweeteners. Clover is a legume, so that clover honey might affect a person sensitive to legumes. Health food stores usually have several different kinds of honey so that anyone who could tolerate honey at all could find a suitable type, perhaps tupelo, avocado or eucalyptus honey, to name just some possibilities. To keep from becoming sensitive to the bee-element in honey, it would be a good idea to rotate it with other sweeteners. One alternative is carob syrup, not the chocolate-like kind, but a clear amber syrup which resembles honey. Carob is in the legume family. Cane sugar and beet sugar could be used on different days.

HOW TO CONTROL YOUR ALLERGIES

There are a number of different oils to choose from and their family classifications should be considered also, both with regard to other foods in the meal and rotating so that no one oil is used too frequently. Obviously one's sensitivities need to be taken into account also; a person sensitive to walnuts, for instance, had best avoid walnut oil. Read the label of margarines to find out the kind of oils used. With salad dressings both oils and sweeteners need to be taken into account. Practically all supermarket salad dressings contain corn sweeteners, and usually corn oil too. Vinegar, used in many salad dressings, may be either apple cider vinegar (apple family) or white vinegar (cereal grass family). Certain spices or flavorings may affect some people. You may prefer to make up your own dressings.

Table I
Plant Food Families Alphabetically
According to Name of Food

Food Name	Family	Food Name	Family
alfalfa	legume	asparagus	lily
almond	plum	avocado	laurel
allspice	myrtle	banana	banana
anise	parsley	barley	cereal
apple	apple	basil	mint
apricot	plum	bay leaf	laurel
arrowroot	single	beans	legume
artichoke,	composite	beet	beet
common or		blackberry	rose
globe		blueberry	heather
artichoke,	composite	boysenberry	rose
Jerusalem		brazil nut	single

Note: Foods designated as "single" have no other foods in that family.

Food Name	Family	Food Name	Family
broccoli	mustard	cranberry	heather
Brussels sprout	mustard	cucumber	gourd
buckwheat	buckwheat	currant	gooseberry
butternut	walnut	dandelion	composite
cabbage	mustard	date	palm
cantaloupe	gourd	dewberry	rose
caraway	parsley	dill	parsley
carob	legume	eggplant	potato
carrot	parsley	elderberry	single
cashew	cashew	endive	composite
cauliflower	mustard	escarole	composite
cayenne	potato	fennel	parsley
celery	parsley	fig	mulberry
celery cabbage	mustard	filbert	single
chard, Swiss	beet	garlic	lily
cherry	plum	ginger	ginger
chestnut (not inc. water ch.)	single	ginseng	single
		gooseberry	gooseberry
chicory	composite	grape	single
chili	potato	grapefruit	citrus
chives	lily	green pepper	potato
chocolate	stercula	guava	myrtle
cinnamon	laurel	hazelnut	single
citron	citrus	hickory	walnut
clove	myrtle	hop	mulberry
cocoa	stercula	horehound	mint
coconut	palm	horseradish	mustard
coffee	single	huckleberry	heather
cola	stercula	Jerusalem artichoke	composite
collard	mustard		
corn	cereal	kale	mustard
coriander	parsley	kohlrabi	mustard
cottonseed	mallow	kumquat	citrus
cowpea	legume	lambs quarters	beet

HOW TO CONTROL YOUR ALLERGIES

Food Name	Family	Food Name	Family
leek	lily	parsley	parsley
lemon	citrus	parsnip	parsley
lentil	legume	pea	legume
lettuce	composite	peach	plum
licorice	legume	peanut	legume
lime	citrus	pear	apple
litchi (lichi) nut	single	pecan	walnut
loganberry	rose	pepper, black or white	single
macadamia nut	single	pepper, green or red	potato
mace	nutmeg		
malt	cereal	peppermint	mint
mango	cashew	pineapple	single
maple	single	pine nut	single
marjoram	mint	pistachio	cashew
melons	gourd	plantain	banana
millet	cereal	plum	plum
mint	mint	pomegranate	single
molasses	cereal	potato	potato
mulberry	mulberry	prune	plum
mushroom	fungus	pumpkin	gourd
muskmelon	gourd	quince	apple
mustard	mustard	radish	mustard
mustard greens	mustard	raisin (grape)	single
nectarine	plum	raspberry	rose
nutmeg	nutmeg	red pepper	potato
oat	cereal	rhubarb	buckwheat
okra	mallow	rice	cereal
olive	single	rutabaga	mustard
onion	lily	rye	cereal
orange	citrus	sage	mint
oregano	mint	sago	palm
papaya	single	safflower	composite
paprika	potato	salsify	composite

Food Name	Family	Food Name	Family
sassafras	laurel	thyme	mint
savory	mint	tobacco	potato
sesame	single	tomato	potato
sorghum	cereal	tragacanth gum	legume
soybean	legume	triticale	cereal
spearmint	mint	tumeric	ginger
spinach	beet	turnip	mustard
squash	gourd	vanilla	single
strawberry	rose	walnut	walnut
sugar cane	cereal	water chestnut	single
sunchoke	composite	watercress	mustard
sunflower	composite	watermelon	gourd
sweet potato	single	wheat	cereal
	(see note)	wild rice	cereal
tangerine	citrus	wintergreen	heather
tapioca	single	yam	single
taro	single		(see note)
tea	single	yeast	fungus

Note: The true yam is a tropical plant that is in a different family from the sweet potato. The terms yam and sweet potato may be used interchangeably (and inaccurately) in stores and even on the labels of cans. Consider the item to be a yam unless it is clearly labeled otherwise, such as with the designation, "New Jersey Sweet Potato."

Table II
Plant Foods According to Food Family

Apple
apple
pear
quince

Banana
banana
plantain

Beet
beet
chard
lambs quarters
spinach

Buckwheat
buckwheat
rhubarb

Cashew
cashew
mango
pistachio

Cereal
bamboo
barley
corn
millet
oats
rice
rye

Cereal
sorghum
sugar cane
triticale
wheat
wild rice

Citrus
citron
grapefruit
kumquat
lemon
lime
orange
tangerine

Composite
artichoke
chicory
dandelion
endive
escarole
Jerusalem artichoke
  (sunchoke)
lettuce
salsify
sunflower

Fungus
mushroom
yeast

212

Ginger
ginger
tumeric

Gooseberry
currant
gooseberry

Gourd
cantaloupe
cucumber
melons
pumpkin
squash

Heather
blueberry
cranberry
huckleberry
wintergreen

Laurel
avocado
bay leaf
cinnamon
sassafras

Legumes
beans
carob
cowpea
lentil
licorice
peas

Legumes
peanuts
soybean
tragacanth gum

Lily
asparagus
chives
garlic
leek
onion

Mallow
cottonseed
okra

Mint
basil
horehound
marjoram
mint
oregano
peppermint
sage
savory
spearmint
thyme

Mulberry
fig
hop
mulberry

HOW TO CONTROL YOUR ALLERGIES

Mustard
broccoli
Brussel sprout
cabbage
celery cabbage
cauliflower
collard
horseradish
kale
mustard
mustard greens
radish
rutabaga
turnip
watercress

Myrtle
allspice
clove
guava

Nutmeg
nutmeg
mace

Palm
coconut
date
sago

Parsley
anise
caraway
carrot
celery

Parsley
coriander
dill
fennel
parsley
parsnip

Plum
almond
apricot
cherry
nectarine
peach
plum (prune)

Potato
cayenne
chili
eggplant
green pepper
paprika
potato
red pepper
tobacco
tomato

Rose
blackberry
boysenberry
dewberry
loganberry
raspberry
strawberry

Stercula
chocolate
cocoa
cola

Walnut
butternut
hickory nut
pecan
walnut

Single Food Families
Each food in this list is
in a separate food family.
arrowroot
brazil nut
chestnut
coffee
elderberry

filbert (hazelnut)
ginseng
grape (raisin)
litchi (lichi) nut
macademia nut
maple
olive
papaya
pepper (black, white)
pine nut
pineapple
pomegranate
sesame
sweet potato
tapioca
taro
tea
vanilla
water chestnut

Table III
Animal Kingdom Foods Classification

A. *Mammals:* Of mammals commonly considered as food sources each species is different enough to be viewed as a separately family except for the bovines—cattle, buffalo and bison, sheep and goats. Other more exotic ruminants—elk, moose, deer and caribou—are related closely to each other and somewhat more distantly to the bovines.

B. *Birds:* Ordinary food birds may be classified into five families as follows:

1. chicken, pheasant, quail
2. duck, goose
3. grouse
4. guinea hen
5. turkey

The eggs of each family of bird should be considered as equivalent to the meat of the bird itself for rotation purposes.

C. *Seafood and Fresh Water Fishes Classified as Follows:*

Food	Family	Food	Family
abalone	single	crab	decapod
albacore	mackerel	crayfish	decapod
bass (sea)	sea bass	croaker	croaker
bass (lake)	sunfish	drum	croaker
bluefish	single	eel	single
bonito	mackerel	flounder	flounder
bullhead	catfish	grouper	sea bass
carp	single	haddock	cod
catfish	catfish	hake	cod
clam	pelecypod	halibut	flounder
cod	cod	herring	herring

Food	Family	Food	Family
lobster	decapod	sauger	perch
mackerel	mackerel	scallop	pelecypod
menhaden	herring	scrod	cod
mullet	single	sea trout	croaker
mussel	pelecypod	shad	herring
muskelunge	pike	shark	single
ocean perch	single	shrimp	decapod
oyster	pelecypod	silver perch	croaker
perch (fresh water)	perch	skipjack	mackerel
		snapper, red	sea bass
pickerel	(see note*)	sole	flounder
pike, northern	pike	sturgeon	single
pike, walleye	perch (see note*)	sunfish	sunfish
		trout	salmon
plaice	flounder	tuna	mackerel
prawn	decapod	turbot	flounder
red snapper	sea bass	weakfish	croaker
salmon	salmon	whitefish	single

Note: In some areas of the United States the term "pickerel" is used to refer to the walleyed pike; in other areas it refers to a true pike.

Table IV
Fresh Water and Sea Foods According to Family

Decapods
crab
crayfish
lobster
prawn
shrimp

Pelecypods
clam
mussel
oyster
scallop

Cod
cod (scrod)
haddock
hake

Croaker
croaker
drum
sea trout
silver perch
weakfish

Flounder
flounder
halibut
plaice
sole
turbot

Herring
menhaden
sardine*
sea herring
shad

Mackerel
albacore
bonito
mackerel
skipjack
tuna

Sea Bass
grouper
sea bass
red snapper

---

* The term sardine is used commercially to refer to canned herring of various kinds. The specific kind (brisling, sild, etc.) may or may not be indicated on the label, but each may be considered a separate variety within the same family. Note the type of oil or sauce they come in.

Fresh Water Species
Catfish
bullhead
catfish

Perch
sauger
walleye
yellow perch
pickerel (see note)

Pike
pickerel (see note)
northern pike
muskellunge

Salmon
salmon species
trout species

Sunfish
black bass species
bluegill

crappy
sunfish

Single Food Families
Each food in this list is
in a separate family
abalone
anchovy
bluefish
carp
eel
lake whitefish
mullet
ocean catfish
ocean perch (rosefish)
shark
smelt
squid
sturgeon
swordfish
tilefish
whitefish

References

1. United States Department of Agriculture, Handbook No. 8, *Composition of Foods*, Washington, D.C., 1963, p. 51.

2. Rinkel, Herbert J., M.D., Randolph, Theron, G., M.D., and Zeller, Michael, M.D., *Food Allergy*, Charles C. Thomas, Springfield, Illinois, 1951, p. 237.

3. ibid., p. 240

4. ibid., pp. 63-4

CHAPTER 10

Living With
Your Allergies

THE MAIN THEME running through this book has been
detecting allergens and avoiding them. This may very well
involve giving up some of one's favorite foods; indeed, they
may have been favorite *because* of the allergy-addiction
phenomenon. Doing what is necessary to avoid allergens
can put a severe wrench in one's life. I pass by many foods
in the supermarket that I genuinely enjoyed in the past and
have to tell myself that they are no longer for me. We get
emotional associations with foods that are tied to family
events, social occasions, feelings, etc. so that making
changes in foods is more than just a matter of nutrition.
Aside from this, there can be problems raised by eating
away from home; travel and eating in restaurants or even at
the homes of friends is likely to confront one with allergens.
The difficulties will be different for each individual
depending on the number and strength of his or her
sensitivities.

In this chapter we will look at some things which should
help to make the life of the allergic person at least a little bit
easier. You may even discover some new foods which you

will like far better than your old ones and conclude, as I have at times, that the life of a person with allergies is not such a deprived one after all. Unless your limitations are very severe, you should be able to enjoy a very satisfying diet from the standpoint of both nutrition and taste.

It is heartening to think that allergy families have an easier time today in most places than they did prior to the 1970s. A greatly increased public concern has led to the spread of health food stores throughout the country, even into many smaller sized communities. People with special dietary needs can have a much easier time meeting them than before. Those sensitive to wheat may be able to tolerate other grains and can find wheat-free breads, and flours from a variety of grains and other foods. Milk-sensitive individuals can get soybean substitutes. Persons who are sensitive to the chemicals on foods have an easier time getting organically grown unsprayed fruits and vegetables. Parents following the Feingold diet can find additive-free frankfurters, cookies, etc. A word of caution is in order though; even some brands of prepared foods sold in health food stores may contain artificial colors or flavors, so one must still read the label.

A person with allergies needs to be conscious of diet and nutrition for two reasons. First, in avoiding the foods to which one is sensitive, a person also bypasses the nutrition that is contained in those foods. If they are important foods which have made a major contribution to the person's diet, then he or she must make sure their equivalent nutrient value is provided in some other way. This is mainly a matter of maintaining one's general level of health. For a person with allergies this is an important consideration, because a higher overall level of health will better enable one to handle the stresses, even if only occasional or accidental, that allergy produces. Second, it may be that the allergic person could benefit from additional nutritional supplements, in some cases extending into the megavitamin range. We will take a look at both of these factors here.

Dietary Supplementation

Some people have found that allergic reactions have been reduced or even eliminated through the use of vitamins, chiefly vitamin C and some of the vitamins in the B-complex family. B vitamins mentioned particularly in connection with allergy are B3, B6, pantothenic acid, and B-15 (pangamic acid). The latter is relatively new, somewhat controversial and not available everywhere. The others have been well established for years and may be safely taken in quantities far larger than the Recommended Dietary Allowances. Whether the vitamins will help in any particular case and the quantities needed will be highly variable for each individual and can only be determined through personal experimentation. Ideally, this should be done under the supervision of a nutritionally oriented doctor. If such a physician is not available in one's community, a person could rely on a book for guidance such as H. L. Newbold's *Mega-Nutrients for Your Nerves* (Peter Wyden Publishers, New York) or Richard Passwater's *Supernutrition* (Dial Press, New York). The basic principle is to experiment with different vitamins at different levels of consumption until one finds the amounts that produce the greatest feeling of well-being. One reason vitamins may not be effective for some people or may be required in very large amounts is that the same defect which causes the allergy symptoms may interfere with the body's ability to absorb and utilize the vitamin itself.[1]

Although vitamin and mineral needs can be highly variable from one person to another, and each person will need to determine his or her needs through varying the amounts taken and noting the effects, we can get an indication of the possible range and kinds of nutrients needed from a paper by Philpott. He states:[2] "A proposed optimum supernutrition program is on this order.

Vitamin C—2-4 grams three times a day. Powder is the best tolerated. Calcium ascorbate has the highest tolerance.

B6—100-500 mg. three times a day.

B5(pantothenic acid) 100-500 mg. three times a day.

B2—100-500 mg. three times a day.

B1—100-500 mg. three times a day.

B3—500-1,000 mg. three times a day either as niacin or niacinamide.

PABA—100-500 mg. three times a day.

L-Glutamine—100-500 mg. three times a day.

Vitamin E—200-800 units three times a day.

Vitamin A—10,000-20,000 units three times a day.

Vitamin D—400-800 units three times a day.

Magnesium as a chelate—75-150 mg. three times a day.

Manganese as a chelate 10-20 mg. three times a day.

Zinc as a chelate—10-20 mg. three times a day.

Such a regimen need not be permanent. Philpott recommends that such large amounts might be needed for only a month or two, as long-standing deficiencies are compensated for, with a reduction possible afterwards. The guide to use in determining how much to cut back is how one feels upon doing so. If a person feels as well with a smaller amount as with a larger then there is no reason for continuing with the larger amount.

Keep in mind that vitamins themselves may be allergenic or that the materials used to prepare the tablets may be. Sensitivity to a vitamin may be checked the same as with foods, either through a sublingual test or by consumption after four days' avoidance. A few people sensitive to corn may react to vitamin C. Most vitamin A is derived from fish oils, so that a person allergic to fish could get a reaction from the vitamin in that form. There are vitamin A preparations made from plant sources, however. People sensitive to cereal grains may react to some types of vitamin E, usually to the oil capsules, the most widely used form of the vitamin. Vitamin E is available in a dry tablet form, however, and this might be better tolerated. Natural vitamin B-complex tablets may contain wheat germ and rice bran.

Philpott also states: "The supplementation of essential amino acids is of prime importance."[3] This is because the poor digestion of protein resulting from pancreatic insufficiency as noted in the preceding chapter usually does not provide the individual with a sufficient amount of all the amino acids needed by the body. Philpott recommends the use of predigested liquid protein—two tablespoons four times a day for a month, then one tablespoon four times a day for the next month, and then on a maintenance basis one tablespoonful twice a day. Amino acid supplementation can result in not just increased tolerance for foods but for inhalants—hydrocarbon fumes, pollen, etc.—as well.

A caution may also be in order regarding predigested liquid protein. The predigestion process is a chemical one similar to that which takes place in the stomach. However, as with natural digestion, traces of the original food may remain and cause reactions in people sensitive to it. So, one needs to keep in mind the possibility of an allergic response to the protein itself. Also, some brands of predigested liquid protein contain artificial colors, flavorings and preservatives which could also affect some people.

Liquid protein has gotten some unfavorable publicity because of some deaths alleged to be due to following a liquid protein diet. However, in these cases the individuals involved ate *nothing but* liquid protein for a long period of time and so had not only a greatly reduced caloric intake but a severely unbalanced diet also. The situation is completely different when liquid protein is taken as a supplement along with other foods normally eaten.

Assisting the Digestion

Based on his findings about allergy and pancreatic functioning, Dr. Philpott has been developing a system for assisting protein digestion which in a number of cases has resulted in decreased sensitivity to allergenic foods to the point where individuals can eat with little or no difficulty foods which otherwise would produce strong reactions. Unfortunately, individuals vary greatly as to their characteristics in this regard and so his approach cannot be reduced to simple standardized instructions. Individual experimentation is required. All I can do here is present the major elements with it being left to the reader to decide if he or she wishes to follow up with this approach and what works best if one does.

In his studies, Dr. Philpott monitored the acidity of the stomach and found this measure to be a useful indicator of patients' reactions to various substances. Although he used more sophisticated means for measuring acidity (e.g., Heidelberg capsule), he says that the degree of the acidity of the stomach is indicated by that of the saliva, which is easy to test. He employs Phydrion (or, more accurately, pHydrion) test paper, although Nitazine paper is equivalent and could be used instead. One or the other should be available at your local pharmacy. A paper with a test range of 4.5 to 7.5 would probably be best initially, although ones with narrower ranges, such as 5.2 to 6.8, are also obtainable. The reading should be made quickly after wetting the paper and in some light other than all-fluorescent.

The test paper is touched to a drop of saliva on the tongue or is dipped in saliva which has been collected in, say, a spoon. The paper will change color according to the pH (degree of acidity or alkalinity) of the saliva. Normal saliva pH is from 6.4 to 6.8—just slightly acid (7.0 is neutral). If the saliva is around 6.8 or higher just before a meal this is an indication that the stomach is not acid enough and that one or two hydrocholoric acid (HCL) tablets should be taken. HCL tablets are available at health food stores. There are two simple cautions which should be observed regarding HCL tablets. They should not be chewed but should be swallowed whole and they should not be taken by anyone with ulcers.

Dr. Philpott's program is based on the use of proteolytic or protein-digesting pancreatic enzymes, supplemented if necessary with bicarbonate. There are a number of different brands of pancreatic enzyme tablets and at least one should be available at your health food store. Potencies may vary somewhat according to brand but each tablet should contain at least between 300 and 400 mg. of pancreas concentrate. Some enzyme tablet formulations also include HCL and are inappropriate for the use described here. They are likely also to be lower in potency in both HCL and enzymes than is recommended by Dr. Philpott. If HCL is needed it should be taken separately, the standard potency for HCL tablets being five grains or 325 mg.

The procedure developed by Dr. Philpott involves taking from one to five enzyme tablets 30 minutes before a meal, one or two HCL tablets just before the meal if a need for this is indicated by testing the saliva, and from one to 10 (although usually five or less) enzyme tablets 30 minutes after the meal, accompanied by alkaline supplementation if indicated by a saliva test made just before the enzyme tablets are taken. If the saliva is below 6.4 one-half hour after finishing a meal "it is a definite indication for a need for alkali supplementation."[4]

LIVING WITH YOUR ALLERGIES

The alkaline supplementation could be frome one quarter to one half teaspoon of sodium bicarbonate (baking soda) mixed in a half-glass of water. Ten-grain sodium bicarbonate tablets may be obtained at a pharmacy, each tablet being equivalent to a quarter-teaspoon. However, an inquiry to one company that makes such tablets, Eli Lilly, resulted in a reply informing me that they also contain starch (of an unspecified kind) and mineral oil. If the starch were made from corn, it could affect a person allergic to that grain and the mineral oil could affect someone sensitive to hydrocarbons. One could avoid these risks and still have a convenient way to provide alkali when away from home and without the need for mixing in a glass by buying empty gelatin capsules and filling them yourself with the sodium bicarbonate. Alkalizer tablets that come in rolls like candy mints contain calcium carbonate rather than bicarbonates and are not recommended by Dr. Philpott.

More effective than sodium bicarbonate, and preferable for those who are restricting their sodium intake, is a mixture of one third potassium bicarbonate and two thirds sodium bicarbonate. As mentioned in the chapter on testing, an approximation to this is available as Alka-Seltzer. However, you could get potassium bicarbonate at a pharmacy or chemical supply house and make up your own mixture. Just be sure the two substances are thoroughly and evenly mixed.

Dr. Philpott has found that allergic reactions to foods are frequently eliminated or reduced in intensity through using this program of enzymes supplemented, if necessary, with HCL and/or bicarbonate. His experience with allergy patients is that they are much more likely to need bicarbonate than HCL. From the allergy theory in the preceding chapter, we can see why this would be so. Only experimentation will show whether enzymes are helpful in a particular case and how many tablets are needed. There seem to be no particular precautions regarding the use of enzymes. As Dr. Philpott notes: "There are no reports of danger in the use of proteolytic enzymes."[5]

The enzymes are made from beef or pork, so it is possible that a person allergic to these foods could have a sensitivity to the enzymes themselves. In my own case, I found that I got a reaction (throat irritation) from a brand of enzymes containing ox bile. The same brand in a formula without the ox bile caused no problems. Those avoiding meat for religious or other reasons might have reservations about using these enzymes. People avoiding only pork could find ones made from beef. Despite his success in using the enzyme program, however, Dr. Philpott still places primary emphasis upon avoidance of allergenic foods, stating that "we should never assume that proteolytic enzyme therapy will be more than a partial answer."[6] He also emphasizes that the person's total life situation should be given attention. Overall stress should be minimized, and one should try for optimum nutrition, exercize, rest, etc.[7]

Delayed Reactions

Delayed reactions to unmasked foods were mentioned in the chapter on testing, but are brought in here, both because they can be quite important in interpreting reactions to specific foods and because the reader now has a broader background of information to focus on them. On the basis of my own experience I would say never to underestimate the possibility of a delayed reaction. It could come during the morning as a result of food eaten the previous day, even near the middle of that day. It could show up sometime after the next meal eaten and so appear to be caused by some food in the latter meal. If you are sure that everything in that meal was safe, then think back to what was consumed earlier—basic food, spice, flavoring or additive. By the same token, carefully test a suspected food to make sure that it really should be avoided and is not being misjudged because of a delayed reaction from an earlier food.

Here is where a diary can be helpful. If it shows a reaction from a food one time but not to that food another time, then the reaction must be due to other foods eaten earlier—assuming that in both cases the food was eaten between four and 12 days since having it last and that it was eaten in the same form (cooked, raw, dried, etc.)

Testing for saliva pH may be helpful in detecting delayed reactions. I have observed that a delayed reaction which becomes evident during the morning may be signaled by a lower-than-average pH before breakfast. If one suspects a delayed reaction, checks saliva pH and finds it low, then bicarbonate and enzymes taken after the next meal can help to forestall a troublesome reaction. For testing purposes though, you will need to permit enough of a reaction to develop so that you can be sure about the food being tested.

Substituting For and
Avoiding Commonly
Allergenic Foods

Whether you are avoiding a food completely or only part of the time, as when on a rotation diet, there are some foods for which this can be difficult simply because they are so commonly used. We will look at some of them here.

Milk

Milk is one commonly allergenic food which has many uses in cooking and it also is a source of the various kinds of cheeses as well as being used for drinking. Allergy to milk will not in all cases include sensitivity to all types of milk products. Different varieties of cheeses may be tested separately. We need to distinguish allergy to milk and milk products from another condition known as lactose intolerance which in some ways is similar to milk allergy. In the case of lactose intolerance the body either never had or has lost the ability to produce the enzyme lactase, which is necessary in order to digest milk. The milk consumed by a lactose intolerant person will not be digested but will ferment in the intestinal tract, usually producing cramps, nausea and gas, and sometimes also nasal symptoms and anxiety attacks, all two or three hours after the milk has been consumed.[8]

Nonwhites seem to have a much higher incidence of lactose intolerance, some groups being as high as two-thirds or more. A lactose intolerant person may be able to consume small amounts of milk with little difficulty but quickly runs into trouble with large amounts. A person might decide, for example, that he or she should be getting more milk for nutritional reasons and increase considerably the amount of milk taken and never realize that the problems which develop are due to the milk. There is evidence that milk intolerant people may actually have a calcium deficiency despite drinking milk because the condition interferes with the absorption of calcium.[9] Fortunately for the lactose intolerants, there is now on the market and available at health food stores a product containing the enzyme lactose which may be taken just before consuming milk that will make normal digestion of milk possible.

For the person with allergy there is no such simple solution. The problem is complicated by the fact that milk is so widely used in so many kinds of foods. A milk-sensitive person should always read the label of prepared foods, "milk solids" or "powdered skim milk" shows up on the label as an ingredient in an amazing number of products. Some people sensitive to milk may be able to tolerate butter, others may not. Only experience will tell for any particular person. As mentioned earlier, ordinary margarines in food stores will contain milk, but "diet" or "imitation" margarines generally do not. These, however, are more like chemical concoctions than food and one should be able to find a more normal margarine not containing milk in health food stores.

Some people who are allergic to cow's milk may have no difficulty with goat's milk, which is becoming more widely available. If fresh goat's milk can not be obtained, then powdered goat's milk may be used. Goat's milk also is made into a number of different types of cheeses ranging from a dark strong-flavored type to light mild varieties. Goat's milk ice cream is also made. A word of caution might be in order though. A person sensitive to cow's milk should probably not eat goat's milk or its products too frequently in order to prevent developing a sensitivity to them.

Another alternative to either cow's milk or goat's milk (and much less expensive and more widely available than the latter) is soy milk. It will not have the same taste, appearance, or "mouth feel" as ordinary milk but when one accepts it in its own right it can be very palatable and useful. Use one cup of soy powder (not soy flour) to a quart of water and mix briefly in a blender with a little sweetening added to give a more palatable flavor. While the soy product may then be used directly it is improved both in taste and in nutritional qualities by being cooked for 20 minutes in a double boiler, stirring occasionally during the time.

For quite some time I resisted the cooking because of the extra time and trouble it took, but after trying the cooked product I quickly concluded it was well worth the extra effort. Cooked soy milk is thicker in consistency and has less of a tendency to settle than the uncooked. Settling may be further reduced by adding a tablespoonful of lecithin to the milk during the mixing. Do not try to get by without using a double boiler even if you use very low heat on an electric stove or you will have a very difficult pan-cleaning job afterward. I know from experience! You can reduce the number of times you need to cook the soymilk by making it more concentrated when you prepare it and then mixing the concentrate with water to give the proper consistency for use. Two cups of soy powder to one quart of water will be accommodated by most double boilers and will be enough for two quarts of finished soy milk. Both the soy milk and the concentrate will keep for up to a week in the refrigerator.

Soy milk can be used as a replacement for cow's milk in most foods. It works very well in dishes such as creamed tuna fish or creamed chicken. Soybean tofu, broken up into little pieces with a fork, provides an approximation to cottage cheese. With any soy product used as a substitute for milk it should be kept in mind that the nutritional values are not strictly equivalent. While soy is high in protein it is not as well balanced in amino acids as is milk and it contains only a fraction of the calcium of milk.[10] While a quart of cow's milk will supply the full daily requirement of calcium, soy milk contains only about one-sixth as much. Either other calcium-rich foods should be eaten or a calcium dietary supplement should be taken if soy milk is used.

Substitutes for ordinary milk may also be made using nuts or seeds including almonds, cashews, sesame and sunflower either singly or in combinations. A proportion of about one cup of nuts or seeds to one quart of water is a good starting point, but you may wish to vary them somewhat according to your personal taste. Mix at a high speed in a blender for two or three minutes. You may wish to strain the milk afterward to eliminate the more chewy particles, using what is strained out on cereals or in baking. It is all highly nutritious. Cashews give a mild flavor and creamy texture either alone or mixed with other ingredients. As an introduction to nut milks, try either two thirds almonds and one third cashews or half sunflower seeds and half cashews. Of course, neither the seeds nor nuts should have been salted before use.

Sweeteners

The whole matter of deserts and sweets raises the question of sweetening, some aspects of which have been mentioned already. From everything we know about sugar-containing foods, it is clear that they should be eaten with much moderation. But moderation does not mean abstinence, and some types of sweetening will be used by practically everyone. Of the two types of common sugar, beet and cane, we have seen that people allergic to beets may be sensitive to beet sugar and that sugar cane is a member of the cereal grass family and hence might provoke a reaction in someone sensitive to cereal grains. We should also remember that raw sugar, brown sugar, turbinado sugar, molasses and sorghum, all of which are preferred over white sugar by health-conscious people, are also all derived from the cereal grasses. Thus, while the idea may be heretical from the standpoint of the health movement, white beet sugar may be preferable to raw cane sugar for the person who can tolerate beets but not the cereal grasses.

With any refined product there is the possibility that materials used in the processing itself may introduce an allergenic component. Thus, Randolph reports on cases of people with chemical sensitivities who also got reactions from cane sugar.[11] Analyzing the sugar production process, he concluded that bone char, through which cane syrup was filtered, was transferring hydrocarbons to the syrup, the hydrocarbons having been absorbed from an open gas flame over which the bone char had been heated previously.

The person buying prepared foods in a restaurant or supermarket of course has no way of knowing what kind of sugar has been used in a particular item. The label on a product need only say "sugar," and manufacturers may change back and forth between beet and cane as market conditions vary. One man, allergic to beet sugar, cautiously tested a certain brand of catsup (ordinary catsup is almost 30% sugar) and found it safe. A bottle of the same brand bought at the same store a month later gave him a reaction. The manufacturer had gotten a good buy on a batch of beet sugar and had used it instead of cane in the catsup contained in the second bottle the man bought.[12] Probably even more commonly used in prepared foods and more likely to affect a larger number of people than beet or cane are the corn-derived sweeteners (corn syrup, dextrose, etc.). The possibility of three kinds of sweeteners means that the consumer faces what Randolph calls a "trilemma" in which reading the labels is not even very helpful.

Although sensitivity to sugars was reported as far back as 1926, it has only been in more recent years that a realization of the extent of allergy to sugars has been recognized.[13] Conventional thinking was that only proteins could cause allergy. Also, dextrose and glucose are produced naturally within the body and it was thought that corn dextrose and glucose were no different from the human products and hence could not cause trouble. Not only have these beliefs turned out to be false, but it has been found that corn sugars "are particularly effective in carrying the allergenicity of corn."[14]

Beet sugar is also a "potent allergen," both with regard to the ease with which sensitivity to it develops and the severity of symptoms which can develop from it.[15] It has been found that consuming cane sugar or corn-derived sweeteners during the four day avoidance period prior to a feeding test can maintain the masking for cereal grasses and thus prevent their detection as allergens. Beet sugar can similarly continue the masking for beets.[16] This material on sugar sensitivity helps to underscore the warning given earlier that if you are being given medical treatment, particularly in a hospital, you should let your doctor know if you have a corn sensitivity in case he intends to administer a dextrose intravenous solution.

The safest course for someone with a sugar sensitivity is to avoid prepared foods, the sweetening source of which is not clearly stated. This is likely to mean making things at home from scratch. The person who can tolerate cane can use raw or turbinado sugar and molasses. Someone who is sensitive to cane will have to settle for beet sugar or other sweetenings. Two guides to use in the supermarket are that beet sugar is ordinarily produced in either the mountain or midwest parts of the country and is simply labeled "sugar." Cane sugar generally comes from the east and west coast areas and is generally labeled as cane sugar.

There are a number of other possibilities for sweeteners besides simple sugar. Honey is the most common, but health food stores are likely to have such other sweeteners as date sugar, maple sugar and maple syrup, carob syrup, etc. While these are all considerably more expensive than ordinary sugar they also have some nutritional value as compared with sugar. Besides, you should not be using so much of any type of sweetening that cost is a major factor. Your health food store will also have brands of prepared foods such as catsup and salad dressings which are sweetened with honey rather than sugar, thus avoiding the problem of wondering whether a product contains cane, beet or corn.

There is, of course, the possibility of artificial sweeteners, but these can have their own problems. At the time of this writing the most common one is saccharin, but it is suspect as a possible producer of cancer and its availability may be restricted in the future. Other sweetener products may become common in the future. As with the natural sweeteners, a person may have sensitivities either to the substance from which a product is made, or to chemicals used in the manufacturing process. A person with chemical sensitivities should be particularly cautious about artificial sweeteners.

Other Substances

Eggs can be a problem because they are not just eaten by themselves but are frequently employed both for their flavor and because they have mechanical qualities that affect the texture or structure of food mixtures containing other ingredients. Thus, egg acts as a binder for ground meat in meat loaves and meatballs. Most health food stores have a product called egg replacer which has many of the binding and thickening characteristics of eggs. Do not confuse this with the no-cholesterol egg substitute products in supermarkets which contain egg white, the part of the egg people are most likely to be sensitive to. A paste made of soaked dried apricots blended and strained can be kept in the refrigerator and used as an egg replacer in many dishes.

Anyone sensitive to milk will find that common types of chocolate are ruled out because they contain milk. In addition, there are the many people who are allergic to chocolate itself. For those of us who like the flavor of chocolate, providence has been kind in providing carob, a food unrelated to chocolate which nevertheless has a flavor similar to it and can be used in many of the same ways. Of course, there seems to be no food to which some people are not sensitive and so carob cannot be thought of as safe for everyone, but many people who cannot tolerate chocolate have no trouble with carob. It is in the legume family so that those who are sensitive to peas, beans, etc. should be cautious about it, and even if they find they can tolerate carob should not eat it every day lest a reaction to it develop.

As a powder, carob can be used like cocoa in baking and in making beverages, possibly with soy milk or with nut milks; as a solid it can be used the same way as chocolate. Most carob prepared like milk chocolate does contain milk, but it should be possible to buy through your health food store bulk bars or chunks of milk-free carob. These contain turbinado sugar, however, which could affect some people. If this form of carob can be tolerated it may be eaten either directly as a candy or melted in a double boiler or in a container set in hot water and used in a variety of ways, such as mixing with peanuts to make a confection or as a coating on a nut and dried fruit mixture. Adding a little coconut oil to the melted carob makes it somewhat softer after it has cooled. Aside from allergy considerations, carob has a number of nutritional advantages over chocolate.

Soymilks and nutmilks can be used in making ice cream types of desserts. While anyone with allergies should go easy on sweets as pointed out earlier, a moderate amount of a desert containing nutritious ingredients in addition to the sweetening should certainly be possible for most people. Ice cream freezers for home use are moderate in price and the process of using them is not difficult. With a little extra freezer space available you can make and store extra icecubes for the ice cream maker. The *Ten Talents* cookbook, to be described later, has recipes for a variety of frozen desserts not using milk.

The person allergic to some cereal grains will find that there are many possibilities for flours. Despite the genetic similarity of wheat, rye and barley, a number of wheat-sensitive people may be able to tolerate one or both of the others. In addition to oat, rice and millet flours, which are in the cereal grain category, there are buckwheat, soy and potato flours. To avoid developing new sensitivities it would be good to rotate the use of these so as to not to have too much exposure to any one. Rye flour can give a rather light texture to baked foods if enough baking powder is used; my wife uses 2½ teaspoons to one cup of flour. A number of different flours can make good gravies.

A substitute for cereal grain flours in baking can be a mixture of two parts of soy flour to one part of potato starch (not potato flour). Packages of Cellu brand soy flour (packed by Chicago Dietetic Supply, Inc., La Grange, Illinois 60525) contain a folder giving recipes for breads using this mixture. Cellu brand soy flour is rather coarse ground and breads made from it are somewhat light and delicate. Other brands of soy flour which are more finely ground produce a more solid heavier loaf which does not rise as well, but also is not as crumbly. With the yeast bread, dough that rises too much has a tendency to fall during the baking. Experimentation and possibly mixing finer and coarser kinds of soy flour could give you practically any type of texture that you would wish. With a little extra sweetening this bread would make a good substitute for cake. Substituting a quarter cup of carob powder for an equivalent amount of the dry ingredients would give you a loaf with a chocolate-like flavor. Either tapioca flour or arrowroot flour may be substituted for potato starch and used in combination with soy flour in these and other recipes.

Some people are sensitive not to the food but to the container in which it is stored or cooked. Chemically sensitive people may be affected by the plastic lining in some types of tin cans but will be able to eat the same kind of food packed in a glass container.[17] I have never heard of anyone being allergic to glass. For some people iron or aluminum cooking utensils may be culprits. Glass and porcelain-enamel utensils would be safe for them and probably stainless steel also. Plastic containers for foods, plastic food wrapping, and plastic food packages can also cause trouble for some people. An alternative, old-fashioned wax paper, of course contains a hydrocarbon and would not be satisfactory for some people. As with plastics generally, the less of an odor a plastic wrap or container has the less likely it would be to cause trouble.

You may find, in the course of avoiding incriminating foods in your diet that you develop new sensitivities. RRZ generally imply that these result from additional exposure to formerly innocent foods. Coca, however, provides an alternative explanation with his distinction between major and minor allergens. The major allergens are the ones that are discovered upon initial testing. When these are eliminated from the diet some people eventually develop symptoms again and it is found that there are other things they are allergic to. It is these which Coca calls the minor allergens, his explanation being that the person's sensitivity to them is of such a low order that their effect is covered up by the presence of the more "powerful" major allergens.[18]

This is not the same thing as masking, which refers to an already-existing allergy having its effects obscured by a partial adaptation to it by the body. A minor allergen does not even become active until the major allergens have been eliminated from the diet. I recently had a strong reaction after eating some watermelon one afternoon. I had had some only once, about a month earlier, since the preceding summer so that it was not a case of heavy exposure leading to sensitivity. In earlier years I had no trouble from watermelon. The only conclusion I can draw is that it is a minor allergen which only became evident after I started avoiding my major ones—milk, eggs and most of the cereal grains.

Unfortunately, hobbies and other recreational activities should not be overlooked in the search for allergens in the contact or inhalant categories. Woodworking means odors from the wood itself, sawdust and various chemicals in adhesives and finishing materials. Modelmaking, arts and crafts involve exposure to plastics, solvents, paints, dyes, etc. Outdoor activities can take one to where fields have been sprayed with hydrocarbon insecticides and weed-controlling chemicals. A person might well decide to court some discomfort in pursuit of an enjoyable hobby but at least he or she should know where the trouble would be coming from.

Perhaps the reader has already wondered why, if reactions to an allergen are masked, one simply cannot continue to eat the allergenic food and rely on masking to control the symptoms. We need to take into account, however, that there are two types of symptoms. First, are those that can develop shortly after eating the food, as when testing it after at least four days of avoidance. It is these symptoms which can be suppressed through masking, which develops from eating the food every day or so. The second type of symptom results when the body can no longer handle the stress of eating an allergenic food and stage III of the G.A.S. is reached.

symptom through masking, the body still is being stressed by the food and adaptation can break down at any time resulting in development of symptoms of the second type, that is, one or more of any of the dozens of illnesses that can be caused by allergy. However, some people might be able to eat a stressor food with symptoms of the first type being controlled by masking and symptoms of the second type held off through adaptation of the body.

Most clinical ecologists do not discuss this possibility, but RRZ mention it briefly and say that it might be possible to produce an absence of symptoms through controlled masking. They say: "It is possible to mask perfectly only a few foods in a given patient, but when feasible, it appears to be desirable in most respects."[19] In this case the person would eat the food once every day or so to maintain the masking. Anyone doing this should realize though, that the absence of symptoms is at the expense of body stress (stage II of the G.A.S.) and that at any time the adaptation can wane and symptoms of the second type can develop. In this event, the person would then have to start avoiding the food.

Even though controlled masking might work for some people there is little in the literature to support this course of action. I believe that most clinical ecologists would prefer that their patients avoid a stressor food. In the majority of cases avoidance would result in losing sensitivity to it, so that the person could then resume eating it on a not-too-frequent basis.

We have seen that for the majority of people, allergies are not fixed permanently but can come and go depending upon the degree of exposure to different foods over a period of time. This means that one will not test for food allergies once, engrave them upon stone, and then be able to consider the job done for a lifetime. Many people will have a need to check their current status from time to time to see if old sensitivities have been lost or new ones have developed.

As you find out which allergies are permanent and which are cyclical for you, and how often you can safely eat foods which are cyclical allergens, your need for testing should decrease sharply, but you will always have the basic principles and methods available any time you wish to use them. Once you have gotten the "lay of the land" from your initial testing, checking foods later on will be much easier. You will have found out which foods are trouble-free for you and will have worked out a diet which is generally satisfactory. Checking on one particular food after that will be much simpler because you can just be sure you do not eat any of it for four days and then have a test meal of it without the need to drastically change your eating patterns. Your other foods will be known quantities, and if there is a doubt you can make another test after four days.

The possibility of allergy tends to be overlooked even within the health food movement. Books and articles on health foods constantly urge the use of wheat germ, bran (which has gotten even more attention lately with the increased interest in roughage in the diet), whole wheat bread and yogurt. Many protein products contain milk and egg. These are all wonderful foods *for those who are not sensitive to them*, but they are among the most allergenic foods there are. An allergy-prone individual should approach them with great caution, testing them carefully to be sure they are innocent before eating them. Even then one should remember that sensitivities can be acquired as a result of too-frequent exposure which can turn foods into offenders, possibly with their reaction masked. Such foods may not be for you.

In trying to get enough to eat while at the same time avoiding my allergens, I have experimented with a number of foods and food combinations that are out of the ordinary. I have found it possible to make "pancakes" out of a variety of things. None of them have the light texture and golden-brown color of ordinary pancakes, but all of them I find quite satisfactory, usually for breakfast. My favorite is a mixture of equal amounts of lentil flour and tapioca flour plus at least a teaspoon of baking powder for every cup of dry ingredients and enough water to give a proper consistency. Up to a tablespoon of oil may be added if desired. They should be cooked on a griddle at about 250° and can be eaten with butter or margarine and honey, maple syrup, or carob syrup just like ordinary pancakes. We have a crank-type flour mill which I use to grind my own lentil flour, but it might be possible to buy lentil flour some places.

A high-protein pancake can be made with approximately equal parts of nutritional yeast and potato starch or tapioca or arrowroot flour, also with baking powder and possibly oil added. There are a number of mild-flavored, good-tasting nutritional yeasts on the market, at least some of which should be available at your health food store.* A mixture of two parts soy flour and one part potato starch plus baking powder is another possibility. Buckwheat flour pancakes are another alternative. By using different ingredients on different days one can still follow a rotation diet. I find it amusing that I, whose favorite food was pancakes, never eat them any more but can still have "pancakes" almost every day without ever touching wheat flour, eggs or milk.

A note about baking powder. Commercial baking powders may contain corn starch. Check the label. You can make your own baking powder by mixing together well one part potassium bicarbonate, two parts cream of tartar and two parts arrowroot flour.

* People who are not used to nutritional yeast may find that it causes intestinal gas. If you have not used it regularly before it would be a good idea to start with a teaspoon or so in a glass of juice the first day and gradually increase the amount of yeast over a period of time. I can have a cup of yeast at a time with no problem whatever resulting from it.

Stir-Fry Cooking

People who are only marginally sensitive to some foods may benefit from having them cooked using the stir-fry technique. With this method foods are cooked quickly in a small amount of oil in a hot utensil. The oil slows down the absorption rate of the food by the body and can space it out enough so that no reactions develop. The stir-fry technique is basically the same as that used by the Chinese in much of their cookery using the wok.

In wok cookery the cooking time is brief, usually just a few minutes. The food is cut into small sized pieces just before cooking, at a minimum temperature at 350°. The fats or oils used must be capable of withstanding the temperature and in accordance with the principles of a rotation diet, different oils should be used on different days. While the high temperatures lend themselves better to cooking with gas, electric stir-fry cooking is quite feasible and electric woks are available. Health food stores are likely to have both recipe books describing the wok method of cooking and woks themselves. This method of cooking has benefitted many people and is certainly worth exploring.

Aids in Cooking and
Meal Planning

The number and kind of particular allergens that different people might be sensitive to is so varied that no specific suggestions can be given here. What I can do is suggest some sources which might prove useful, primarily to those who have sensitivities to one or more of the basic foods used in the American diet—corn, wheat, eggs, milk, beef, etc.—which as we have seen are the foods which are most commonly allergenic. There are a number of books containing food information and recipes using other than the usual ingredients which would be of particular value to those with the most common allergies. These are:

Ellen Buchman Ewald, *Recipes for a Small Planet*, Ballantine Books, New York, A companion volume to *Diet for a Small Planet*, it contains high protein meatless recipes for hot dishes, breads and cereals, and desserts. Soybeans are stressed but some recipes also call for egg, milk and cheese.

Frank J. Hurd, D.C. and Rosalie Hurd, B.S., *A Good Cook ... Ten Talents*, published by the authors, Box 86A, Route 1, Chisholm, Minnesota 55719. Contains useful food information as well as many recipes for main dishes, breads and cereals, soups, salads and salad dressings, etc. practically all of which use neither meat, milk, nor eggs. Excellent for those needing to avoid such foods.

El Molino Mills, *El Molino Best Recipes*, Alhambra California, 91803. A durable little book put out by a producer of specialty foods. Contains recipes using carob (a nutritious substitute for chocolate) and a section with allergy recipes in addition to a variety of other recipes.

Hanna Kroeger, *Allergy Baking Recipes*, Johnson Publishing Co., Boulder, Colorado, 80302. A small book with mostly baking recipes which do not use one or more of the common allergens. Each ingredient is listed in capital letters so that you can quickly tell if any particular recipe calls for a food which is being avoided.

Frances Moore Lappé, *Diet for a Small Planet*, Balantine Books, New York. Provides very valuable information for vegetarians about getting adequate protein in the diet by eating nutritious combinations of plant foods. Does not try to avoid milk, wheat, and eggs.

Mothey Parsons, *Almonds to Zoybeans*, Larchmont Books, New York. A good collection of vegetarian recipes covering a range of types of foods—soups, main dishes, beverages, etc.—with the emphasis on good protein nutrition. Does not try to avoid milk, wheat, and eggs.

United States Department of Agriculture, *Baking for People with Food Allergies*, Washington, D.C., 1976, 35¢. A sixteen page booklet. It is usually much faster to order through your Congressman than through the Government Printing Office.

Three books deserve special mention because they have been prepared from the standpoint of clinical ecology. The first, *Very Basically Yours: An Allergy Cookbook*, was compiled by June Larson and Bonnie Nugent and may be ordered from: Mrs. Bonnie Weidman, 5460 North Marmora Avenue, Chicago, Illinois 60630. The book is a project of the Human Ecology Study Group, which consists primarily of patients of Dr. Randolph. In addition to recipes avoiding the common allergens, the book also has information on substances contained in common prepared foods, information on stir-fry cooking, and food classification tables.

The second book is *Management of Complex Allergies: The Patient's Guide* by Natalie Golos, published by the New England Foundation for Allergic and Environmental Diseases, 3 Brush Street, Norwalk, Connecticut 06850. The foundation was established by Dr. Marshall Mandell. In addition to recipes, the book also has information on sources of supply for exotic meats (elk, moose, etc.) and uncommon clothing materials. It also contains material useful to someone with chemical sensitivities.

Finally, there is the *Allergy Handbook* by Kay Ludeman and Louise Henderson available through Human Ecology Research Association, 12110 Webb Chapel Road, Plaza III, Suite E305, Dallas, Texas 75234. It has extensive food tables which include many herbs and spices, and over a hundred recipes. It also deals with chemical sensitivities and has recommendations for alternatives to toiletry or cosmetic items to which individuals might be sensitive.

A Final Personal Note

When I had first learned of clinical ecology and did my initial testing of the foods I had been eating most frequently, I found out that I was sensitive to milk, wheat and eggs. Even during the course of writing this book though, I have uncovered previously unsuspected sensitivities. In the case of at least one food, peanut, I believe that this developed from eating it too frequently as I cut out other foods from my diet. After avoiding peanut for a few months I have been able to go back to it, but limit its consumption to about once a week, eating other legumes in between. While I might be able to tolerate eating peanut more frequently, I would rather follow my present schedule than risk a resensitization requiring another period of avoidance. My experience confirms the cautions of clinical ecologists that a person with some allergies should not eat any one food too often lest a sensitivity to it develop.

I have had to change my conception of myself from being a person who could eat anything to being someone who had to watch out for only a few specific foods, and finally I have had to realize that I have many sensitivities (cereal grains, many kinds of nuts, most fruits, and some kinds of fish and fowl) calling for careful regulation of my diet. Fortunately I have no trouble with ordinary meats and vegetables, but I also eat these on a rotation basis because I certainly do not want to develop any more sensitivities. I still get reactions at times, either from trying out new foods, or more commonly now, from ingredients in incidental foods (salad dressings, sauces, etc.) eaten away from home.

Is having to be so concerned about diet inconvenient?

Yes. Do I wish it were otherwise? Definitely. Is it worth it to me so that I can avoid the kinds of troubles I had in the past? Most emphatically. I view my situation as something like that of a diabetic in that constant concern with one's diet is required. It would be nice to be able to eat anything at any time, but for me, and perhaps for you, it is simply not possible to do without suffering unpleasant consequences.

Throughout all my testing and experimenting with my diet, my wife was very helpful, primarily with moral support but also with such useful functions as eating what we had remaining of foods I found I could not tolerate well. She could eat anything with impunity—or so we thought. She had had trouble for years though, with bronchitis or pleurisy attacks and/or pneumonia, almost always occurring in the spring. While a seasonal condition such as this could be caused by a plant pollen inhalent, the variations in timing and symptoms have been so great that this does not appear to be likely.

A particularly serious bout of illness last spring led to our doctor prescribing a type of medication which has the characteristic that its effectiveness is hampered by milk. He warned her then, not to have any milk or other dairy products while taking the medication. Although she did not ordinarily drink milk, she had regularly eaten yogurt and cheese. Simply because milk is allergenic for so many people I suggested that as she had been off of milk products for more than a week while taking the medication, she should view her resumption of them as a test, consuming yogurt all by itself and noting if she detected any reactions afterward, following with a second smaller helping an hour later if nothing developed.

Perhaps more to humor me more than anything else she agreed. Imagine her surprise when shortly after having the yogurt she noticed an unpleasant increase in throat mucus accompanied by coughing, just the kind of coughing that characterized her bronchitis attacks. That was the end of dairy products for her!

Within a few days she started to notice other consequences of giving up milk products. Glands in her neck which had been enlarged to about the size of almonds ever since childhood decreased to a normal pea-size. Post-nasal drip, which was particularly annoying at night, disappeared. Well before this but after I had found and eliminated my major allergens it came as a genuine surprise to me one day when I suddenly realized that my wife was using more tissues for her nose than I was. Now, it is a rare occasion when either of us has need for a tissue.

My wife had another problem, however, which became particularly troublesome during the last year, namely arthritis in her hands. This was despite a nutritious no-nonsense diet and substantial vitamin and mineral supplementation. Then she read an article by Carlton Fredericks reporting on work by Norman F. Childers, Ph.D., a professor of horticulture at Rutgers University.[20] Dr. Childers has compiled data on over 1,200 case histories of arthritics whose condition either cleared up or improved considerably when they avoided foods from the nightshade family—labeled the potato family in the food tables in the preceding chapter.

Short of arthritis, foods in the nightshade family (which also includes tobacco) may cause painful joints and muscles. The older the person is and the more severe the case of arthritis, the longer the period of avoidance that is required in order to produce relief. Dr. Childers says that for some people it may take months, or in extreme cases affecting the elderly, even years of abstinence. My wife's case was just in the beginning stage and she noticed an improvement within just a few days. She has found, though, that even a small amount of a nightshade family food—such as a slice of tomato in a salad—produces a flare-up of symptoms the next day.

I consider her experience quite instructive because here is a case of a person in generally quite good health whom neither of us viewed as having food sensitivities even as I was working on this book, but who now has found two types of foods, dairy products and nightshade family foods, that were trouble-causing for her. As month after month went by without my catching a cold, I found myself thinking that if *I* could go six, then, seven, then eight months without a cold, that almost anyone in the world could do so. By the same token, if my wife can have food sensitivities, then anyone can.

So there you are. I hope that the information given here will be helpful to you and that you will be successful in minimizing problems from allergy.

References

1. Philpott, William H., M.D., *Ecologic Mecicine Manual*, Oklahoma City, Oklahoma, 1975, mimeographed, pp. 20-1.

2. Philpott, William H., M.D., *Ecologic Stimulus Evoked Pancreatic Insufficiency in Chronic Degenerative Disease in General and Cardiovascular Disease in Particular*, Oklahoma City, Oklahoma, mimeographed paper given at International Academy of Metabology, Tucson, Arizona, May 8, 1977, pp. 6-7.

3. ibid., p. 7.

4. ibid., p. 5.

5. ibid., p. 4.

6. Philpott, William H., M.D., *The Significance of Reduced Proteolytic Enzymes in the Diabetes Mellitus Disease Process and in the Schizophrenia Syndrome Variable*, Oklahoma City, Oklahoma, mimeographed paper, April, 1977, p. 3.

7. Philpott, William H., M.D., *Methods of Reversing the Stimuli Evoked Pancreatic Insufficiencies of Chronic Degenerative Diseases*, Oklahoma City, Oklahoma, mimeographed paper presented at the Society for Clinical Ecology, San Francisco, California, October 30, 1977, p. 12.

8. Linda Clark, "Outwitting Food Intolerances," *Let's Live*, August 1977, pp. 19-22; also Philpott, *Manual*, p. 10.

9. Clark, op. cit., p. 20.

10. United States Department of Agriculture *Handbook No. 8*, Washington, D.C., 1963, pp. 39 and 59.

11. Randolph, Theron G., M.D., "The Role of Specific Sugars," in Dickey, Lawrence D., M.D., *Clinical Ecology*, Charles C. Thomas, Springfield, Illinois, 1976, p. 312.

12. ibid., p. 316.

13. ibid., pp. 311-7.

14. ibid., p. 311.

15. ibid., p. 312

16. ibid., p. 317.

17. Randolph, Theron G., M.D., *Human Ecology and Susceptibility to the Chemical Environment*, Charles C. Thomas, Springfield, Illinois, 1962, p. 166.

18. Coca, Arthur F., M.D., *The Pulse Test*, ARC Books, New York, 1959, pp. 169-70.

19. Rinkel, Herbert J., M.D., Randolph, Theron G., M.D. and Zeller, Michael, M.D., *Food Allergy*, Charles C. Thomas, Springfield, Illinois, 1951, p. 242.

20. Fredericks, Carlton, Ph.D., "Your Favorite Foods May Cause Arthritis," *Prevention*, October 1978, pp. 46-48.

Index

A

B

C

INDEX